D0908138

Hunting the 1918 Flu

One Scientist's Search for a Killer Virus

Hunting the 1918 Flu

One Scientist's Search for a Killer Virus

KIRSTY DUNCAN

UNIVERSITY OF TORONTO PRESS
Toronto Buffalo London

© University of Toronto Press Incorporated 2003
Toronto Buffalo London
Printed in Canada

ISBN 0-8020-8748-5

Printed on acid-free paper

National Library of Canada Cataloguing in Publication Data

Duncan, Kirsty
Hunting the 1918 flu : one scientist's search for a killer virus /
Kirsty Duncan.

Includes biliographical references and index.
ISBN 0-8020-8478-5

1. Influenza – History – 20th century.   2. Influenza – Epidemiology.
3. Epidemiology – Moral and ethical aspects.   I. Title.

RC 150.6N67D85 2003   614.5'18'09041   C2002-905704-3

University of Toronto Press acknowledges the financial assistance to its
publishing program of the Canada Council for the Arts and the Ontario Arts
Council.

University of Toronto Press acknowledges the financial support for its
publishing activities of the Government of Canada through the Book
Publishing Industry Development Program (BPIDP).

For my parents,
Helen and Errol Duncan

Contents

Figures

Preface

Reading in 1992 about the horrors of the Spanish flu pandemic of 1918 – healthy adults, for example, dropping dead in mid-activity and putrified corpses lying exposed in deserted streets – and experts' alarming predictions led me to seek answers. Reading Dr Alfred Crosby's book *Epidemic and Peace* inspired me to learn what caused Spanish flu and, in its wake, encephalitis lethargica, or sleeping sickness, a scourge of c.1915–30, which claimed or ravaged the lives of 5 million people.[1]

And after two years of searching for bodies of victims of the Spanish influenza and sleeping sickness that might exist in frozen Alaska, Russia, and Norway, and after extensive correspondence with archaeologists, historians, funeral directors, government officials, and the Lutheran church, I found on Spitsbergen Island the resting place of seven miners, who had all died of Spanskesyken, or Spanish flu, and were buried in permafrost. The frozen ground, I hoped, would have preserved the bodies along with the micro-organism that killed the victims. The miners' graves were marked and had been undisturbed for almost eight decades in Spitsbergen Island, in the province and archipelago of Svalbard, Norway. Small tissue samples from the miners might – despite my own reluctance to disturb the graves – yield fragments of the Spanish influenza virus. The miners might provide the answers to the 1918 pandemic.

I found no victims of sleeping sickness; as a result, the story of encephalitis lethargica largely peters out in the book. I do address the subject, however, as scientific leads sometimes simply disappear, only to reappear later, and also because I hope that someone will take on the challenge of finding its cause and cure.

What follows is my story, the events as I experienced them. This is a key point. I came in contact with over 1,800 people from all walks of life during my nine-year search for the lethal virus. I never met the vast majority of these people face to face; unknown journalists, for example, repeatedly questioned me and often, perhaps after a brief telephone conversation, drifted away, forming their own impressions and making their own judgments about the project and the team.

I worked more closely with approximately 100 people, leading scientists and government bureaucrats from Britain, Canada, Norway, and the United States. My closest contacts were, however, a group of seventeen scientists and professional exhumation specialists who worked in 1998 on the young coal miners in Svalbard. The project was a team effort, and each person brought important and necessary, even vital, expertise – geographical, geological, geophysical, medical, medical-archaeological, microbiological, pathological, and virological.

For nine years, I led the project to determine the cause of the Spanish flu. After finding the resting place of the Norwegian miners, I put together a multinational, multidisciplinary team of experts and spent twenty-two months seeking permission from Norwegian authorities to exhume the miners and to take tissue samples in order to characterize the Spanish flu virus. The team spent two years developing detailed safety protocols and expedition plans for the 1998 exhumations, which yielded over 100 tissue samples. The samples are currently being analysed in Biosafety Level 4 (BSL 4) laboratories, which provide the best possible protection to staff and the environment from deadly pathogens.

It is therefore essential that I properly recognize each and every team member for his or her contribution. I would particularly like to note the outstanding work of the team's Norwegian co-ordinator, Professor Tom Bergan (previously of the National Hospital and University of Oslo), who arranged endless details on the Norwegian side and fought doggedly for recognition of his country's central role in the project.

I base what follows on fifteen four-inch binders containing every fax that I sent and received (I was not privy to every fax in the project) and written accounts of conversations over the entire history of the project, from its conception to today. In addition, I have three volumes of proceedings of workshops and three technical reports.

No other team member could have written this history, as no other person was involved right from the very beginning, during the initial hunt for samples in 1992. Moreover, because of the team's reporting structure, not all members were privy to the great majority of faxes. We had a scientific advisory group (SAG) of six people; five reported to me, the project leader and the sixth member of the SAG, rather than to the whole team. (Three members of the SAG did not even join the project until 1997, five years after it began.) Although the whole team learned of results, some may have been unaware of the difficult negotiations that preceded.

In this book, for easier reading, I group together topics such as scientific planning, development of laboratory agreements, and public relations. Unfortunately, this method obscures the nature of the daily work.

The quotes from faxes and conversations appear in the text in the writers' or speakers' actual words. The majority of conversations were written down (in the presence of a witness) as the telephone conversation took place in my office in my home. Other conversations took place in the presence of a witness or witnesses and were written down immediately afterwards. There were also some in which no witness was present: for example, that with Dr Jeffrey Taubenberger following the 8 April 1997 CDC meeting (see 79–80); I wrote down the conversation immediately. Providing raw data is in keeping with the open dialogue requested by the governor of Svalbard. Correspondence to and from public offices in Norway is open for inspection by everyone, including the press, according to Norway's Freedom of Information Act.

I base chapters 3, 7, 15, and 17 on my experiences and conversations in Norway and, finally, in England and in them cite little correspondence with other team members. These four chapters are, by their very nature, more autobiographical than the rest of the book. I base chapter 15 on four sources – Alan Heginbottom's log book, daily updates for the team's website, Dr Charles Smith's diary, and my nightly records in Longyearbyen.

What emerges is, I believe, a view of science in all its complexity – its dark side and its inspiring side. We see scientists collaborating, competing, and searching for answers. My experience over the past nine years has not been all good, and mine is not an isolated case. Rivalry, covert funding practices, publication wars, and unethical practices do exist in scientific work.

Nevertheless, scientists and science are often shielded from public scrutiny. I hope that my portrait of the Spanish influenza project raises questions about this relatively unexplored territory – the sometimes-unseemly ethics and practice of science.

I also hope that the work raises other questions. For example, how do we weigh medical risks against scientific benefits and costs? How do we establish and define the rights of subjects? What rights do the dead have? How do we balance the rights of subjects with the rights of funders? What agreements should be in place prior to undertaking any study? What are the costs and benefits of media involvement? How do we compare and choose among priorities of different disciplines? How do we limit national agendas in research? I offer no definitive answers, but encourage the reader to think about and to draw his or her own answers and conclusions.

Finally, I hope that this work raises questions about age and gender and how such factors interact with the process of doing science. Science remains personal, despite its reputed neutrality and objectivity, and both ageism and sexism are issues that can no longer be ignored. It has been my experience that young academics and especially female academics, often receive little respect and are, more often than not, used and abused by the system – that is, until they learn to play science's hardball politics.

Acknowledgments

I am grateful to the many people who made possible the search for the 1918 influenza virus in Svalbard, Norway. I am especially grateful for the strong support of the original team members – Mr Alan Heginbottom, Dr Peter Lewin, and Dr Charles Smith – who saw the project through to its fruition and whose initial ideas helped to guide and shape the science. And I am most appreciative of the efforts of Professor Tom Bergan – his commitment, his attention to detail, and his outstanding work on behalf of Norway and the team.

I thank Sensors & Software Inc. for helping the research team undertake the ground-penetrating radar (GPR) study and for analysing the resulting data. I thank the Necropolis Company, whose excellent work the team and I appreciated, for providing the equipment, services, and personnel to enable the scientific team to undertake the exhumations and sampling.

Thank you to committee members of granting councils, members of the scientific establishment, members of the general public, and others who offered assistance and made suggestions and recommendations along the way. In this respect, I would particularly like to thank my colleague and friend Professor Alan Trenhaile, University of Windsor, for his wisdom, guidance, and encouragement during our preparation for the expedition. I also thank the University of Windsor and the University of Toronto for their support.

And finally, I am indebted to the people of Longyearbyen, Svalbard, and Norway, who always made me feel welcome and who treated me with great courtesy and hospitality. I have strong affection for Norway, and I return to the country with eager anticipation and delight. I am pleased that I could record some of the country's beautiful geography and exciting history. I particularly acknowledge, among those who have given me advice and guidance, a past governor of Svalbard, Ann-Kristin Olsen, Pastor Jan Hoifodt, Svalbard Kirke, Mr Kjell Mork, Longyearbyen Skole, and Mr Jan Haugaland of the Norsk Polarinstitutt. And thank you to Ms Ragna Haan, who translated numerous documents for me.

For their help in preparing the manuscript based on the project, I first and foremost thank Mrs Helen Duncan, who edited numerous drafts of every chapter. The following people read the first completed draft of the manuscript: Ms Betty Andriopoulos, Mr Robert Bower, Dr Margaret Helen Rae Brander, Mr Donald Clarke, (previously of Wright and Associates Barristers, Solicitors, Notaries), Mr and Mrs Christopher Duncan, Mr Errol Duncan, Ms Jeannette Marseu, Ms Janine Rosenberg, Ms Marnie Russell, Dr Irving Siegel, Dr Zacharias Suntres, Mr Paul Trudelle (Hull & Hull Barristers and Solicitors), and Ms Patricia Wright (Wright and Associates Barristers, Solicitors, Notaries).

I am especially grateful to Mr Virgil Duff, executive editor, University of Toronto Press, for believing in my book, for his excellent comments, and for his inspiration and insight. I am also grateful to four anonymous referees for their helpful suggestions and particularly to a reviewer for the University of Toronto Press's Manuscript Review Committee, who spent a great deal of time and effort in reviewing and editing the manuscript. And I am thankful to Mr John Parry for his commitment to the book and for his excellent editing skills. It was a delight, honour, and pleasure working with him.

Finally, I am grateful to my husband, Robert Bower, and to my parents, Helen and Errol Duncan, who were with me every step of the way, each and every day.

Hunting the 1918 Flu

Introduction: A Deadly Killer

What follows is the story of Spanish influenza, the great killer and medical enigma of 1918–19, and the search in the frozen reaches of our planet – namely, the town of Longyearbyen, Spitsbergen, Svalbard, Norway – for the virus that caused the disease.

In 1918–19, medical science was at a loss to explain the epidemic of Spanish flu that swept the world in three great waves and killed an estimated 20 million–40 million people in just one year. Medical science was unable to provide sound advice to terrorized populations, who saw many around them dying with spectacular speed and horror. Healthy, robust people might suddenly slump forward or topple over, 'as if struck by lightning'; some died before they ever touched the ground.[1–3]

The cause of the great influenza was unknown, and very few tissue samples from victims were saved for future scientific exploration and possible identification of the lethal virus. As recently as the early 1990s, medical science still had no answers. This despite the fact that influenza is still with us and continues to cause havoc each year. Influenza in fact remains one of the biggest unconquered threats to human health. Every year, outbreaks infect 100 million people in the United States, Europe, and Japan. Each year, influenza infection is responsible for 20–25 million visits to physicians and millions of days lost from work in the United States alone. And every year, the estimated economic cost associated with influenza epidemics in the Northern Hemisphere is $10 billion.[3]

Remarkably, these figures reflect only the regular annual outbreaks of influenza which affect between 10 per cent and 20 per cent of the population. They do not measure the global epidemics, or pandemics, which hit 50 per cent or more of the population. Pandemics, such as those of 1918, 1957, and 1968, usually result in widespread loss of life.[3]

History teaches us that we are due for another fatal flu in the future. The world is much more vulnerable to the eruption and spread of infectious disease today than in 1918, as people tour increasingly, travel more rapidly, and visit many more places than ever before. In fact, few environments on Earth remain truly isolated or untouched.[4]

This dramatic increase in the movement of people means that a person, unknowingly harbouring a life-threatening disease, could board a jet, potentially infect fellow passengers, and be on another continent when his or her symptoms first strike. All those exposed in transit could then pass on the deadly pathogen at their future ports of call. Therefore a health problem in one area of the world could quickly threaten all of Earth's peoples.[4]

Today, even exotic diseases can travel quickly. In 1989, for example, an American man became ill upon returning home from Nigeria, where he attended his parents' funeral. Before being diagnosed with deadly Lassa fever, endemic to most of West Africa, the man came into close contact with 102 people to whom he may have unwittingly passed on the disease before he died.[4]

Perhaps the best-known example of the rapid spread of an infectious disease is that of acquired immunodeficiency syndrome (AIDS), caused by the human immunodeficiency virus (HIV). The global spread of HIV was clearly under way by the mid-1970s. By December 1999, HIV was thought to have killed 16 million people globally.

We must be prepared. The more we know about pandemics – from the molecular structure of their microbes to the ways in which they spread – the greater the probability that we will be able to mitigate their deadly effects – even if they are launched deliberately by human agents.

In North America, the Spanish flu pandemic serves as a useful analogue for the potential ramifications of a major epidemic caused by one of the serious biological weapons, such as *Variola major* (smallpox), *Bacillus anthracis* (anthrax), *Yersinia pestis* (plague), Botulinum toxin (produced by *Clostridium botulinum*), and a number of the causative agents of the syndrome termed viral haemorrhagic fever. Although case fatality rates were 1.9–5.0 per cent for Spanish influenza, they might reach 30–80 per cent for untreated smallpox and anthrax.[5] In the United States, the 1918 influenza pandemic caused 550,000 deaths, widespread social disruption, and enormous burdens on health care and civil infrastructure. A catastrophic epidemic resulting from bioterrorism would 'severely tax society's ability to care for the sick and dying, and to contain disease.' Preparations for any such emergency (for example, pandemic influenza) or bioterrorist attack must therefore include several capabilities – to characterize properly any outbreak, to allocate health resources fairly, to care for mass casualties, and to provide mass burials that respect social codes.[5]

Could Spanish flu reappear? Maybe. Therefore the more we know about it, the better. Finding its cause and describing the causal agent might allow scientists to explain why the disease killed so many and why it disappeared so quickly. Moreover, describing the causal agent might also allow scientists to improve current influenza vaccines and test present anti-viral drugs against the deadly flu.[3]

This book is a study of the search for the 1918 influenza virus, organized into five parts. Part I covers the tracking down of victims of the virus, the development and early evolution of a research team, and my first trip to Spitsbergen. These developments took place between 1992 and June 1997. Part II examines the period around the crucial examination of the burial sites with ground-penetrating radar (GPR), between June and October 1997. In the third part, I trace the complex negotiations and preparations (October 1997–August 1998) for the exhumations. Part IV is the most intense and dramatic phase in the whole story – the three weeks in late August and early September 1998 when we exhumed the flu victims in Spitsbergen and took tissue samples. Part V chronicles the still-unresolved analysis of those samples.

The three phases of our Spitsbergen project – (I) the GPR study of the site; (II) the exhumations; and (III) decoding the virus – correspond approximately with parts II, IV, and V, respectively, of this book.

1 The Spanish Influenza of 1918

The guns fell silent at the eleventh hour of the eleventh day of the eleventh month of 1918. One in ten of those soldiers who had fought in Europe died in the service of his country; an even greater number were wounded in deadly trench warfare. The final cost of the war will never be known. However, estimates of 12 million people dead, 7 million of them soldiers, are almost certainly too low. A total of 3 million people may have died in Russia alone, rather than the usual estimates of 1.7 million there.[1-6]

The war to end all wars was over. 'In one wonderful and joyous explosion, the world went mad.' In most countries, shops closed; throngs of boisterous, jubilant people celebrated in streets; whistles blew, and bands played hit songs such as 'World Peace' – 'From now on, there'll be peace, / They'll wage no war again.' And exhilarated and intoxicated crowds set off fireworks, ignited bonfires, and revelled late into the night.[7] In London, King George V and Queen Mary greeted the crowds from the balcony at Buckingham Palace. The King spoke gratefully; 'With you, I rejoice. Thank God for the victories the Allied armies have won, which have brought hostilities to an end. Peace is in sight.'[8]

Three Waves of Influenza

As the world's peoples were celebrating the end of war, the end of dying, and a fresh beginning, the second and most virulent of three waves of a new killer, 'Spanish influenza,' raged with a ferocity greater than all the killing power of the previous four years of war, killing tens of millions.

Although Spanish flu was new, influenza as such was not. The name 'influenza,' derived from the Italian word for 'influence,' had been used to describe disease beginning in the Middle Ages, when it was believed that illness came from the influence of the stars.[8] The highly contagious, acute respiratory illness known as influenza, however, appears to have afflicted humans since ancient times; Hippocrates recorded one such epidemic in 462 BC. Pandemics of influenza were not new either. They raged in 1732–3, 1775, 1782, 1833, 1836–7, 1847–8, and 1889–90. The pandemic in 1889–90 infected 40 per cent of the world's population, and thousands died.[9] Yet the first wave of Spanish influenza had largely gone unnoticed in the spring and summer of 1918. In fact, the spring wave of the disease did not even receive mention in the index of the 1918 volume of the *Journal of the American Medical Association*.[10] The disease had been mild, the mortality was not unusually high, and the world had been preoccupied with a fifth year of war.[8,10]

However, influenza was brewing quietly, with localized outbreaks in U.S. military camps in early 1918. On 11 March, 107 American servicemen became ill at Camp Funston, Fort Riley, Kansas. By the end of the five-week training camp, 1,127 had been stricken, and 46 had died of pneumonia following the flu. Camps Doniphan, Fremont, Gordon, Grant, Hancock, Lewis, Logan, Kearney, McClellan, Oglethorpe, and others also reported epidemics in March and April.[10]

By April the disease had spread to France – perhaps carried there by American troops.[8] And by the end of April, influenza had reached Spain, where the disease was widely publicized. Neutral Spain had no censorship of its press, unlike countries at war. Spain made the first public announcement of the disease. Madrid cabled London: 'A strange form of disease of epidemic character has appeared in Madrid.'[7,8]

By May it had reached Greece, Macedonia, Egypt, and Britain. In England, 10,313 sailors of the Royal Navy developed flu and were unable to leave port. And the Royal College of Physicians labelled the disease 'Spanish influenza,'[7,8] and the inaccurate name stuck in history. In Britain the disease had been called 'Flanders Grippe'; in Spain, 'Naples soldier'; in Germany, 'Blitz Katarrh,' or lightning cold; and in Switzerland, 'La Coquette,' because it 'passed its favours around so freely.' In Poland it was the 'Bolshevik Disease,' and in Ceylon it was 'Bombay Fever.' In Hong Kong, it was termed 'too much inside sickness.' Perhaps the name 'Spanish flu' persisted because neutral Spain was unpopular with both warring sides, which were hit equally by 'a

foe that cut down troops and sent them behind the lines to first aid stations and hospitals.'[8]

Throughout the spring, there had also been outbreaks on the other
side of the world. Influenza had been reported in China and in March
in the Japanese Navy. By May it was widespread in Asia.[7] Most of the
deaths there were among the elderly, but there were an appreciable
number of deaths among those 20–40 years old.[9]

Second Wave

In the autumn the virus probably mutated, and a worldwide epidemic,
or pandemic, of unprecedented virulence exploded in the same week
in three port cities, thousands of miles apart – Freetown, Sierra Leone;
Brest, France; and Boston, United States. Were they manifestations of
a single mutation of the virus? Did the disease originate in one of
three ports and travel almost instantaneously to the other two? Or
were there different, simultaneous mutations?[10] To date, we have no
answers to these important questions.

The three epidemics launched the autumn wave of Spanish flu and
the most devastating disease outbreak in recorded history in terms of
total mortality. In September, the disease swept Europe. Returning
troops carried flu home. In North America, servicemen disembarked
from crowded ships at Atlantic ports only to board trains that would
take them, along with flu, inland to cities, villages, and farms from
Newfoundland to California.[8]

The second, deadly autumn wave of Spanish flu lasted about six
weeks in each city and then died down. In November, nine days after
the war ended, Cockermouth, England, reported that almost every
family in town was infected following a service of thanksgiving to
peace in the church. A week after the war's end, the number of deaths
in Britain soared to more than 19,000, and the U.S. state of Louisiana
reported 350,000 new cases. By December, a million were sick in Java,
Dutch East Indies, 1,200 were dying daily in Barcelona, Spain, and
250,000 had died in India's Punjab.[7]

Finally, the world took notice. Major nations reported flu in newspapers. One Canadian woman reported that the 'fear was so thick that
even a child could feel it.'[8] Despite the world-wide alarm, most people
developed only a mild flu. Even in the severe autumn wave, 80 per
cent of patients suffered only the usual three-to-five-day illness – initially a cough and stuffy nose, but later a dreadful ache in every joint

and muscle – leaving them feeling as if they 'had been beaten all over with a club,' with a temperature as high as 40°C. If the illness progressed no further, the victim was usually 'back to normal' within a week.[7–11]

But pregnant women recovered more poorly. The prognosis was said to be 'severe' for women who aborted or went into premature labour. One study showed that a total of 26 per cent of 1,350 female victims suffered miscarriage, stillbirth, or premature labour.[9]

Approximately 20 per cent of all influenza patients developed pneumonia. Half of those died. The pneumonia often developed rapidly, with some patients experiencing a 'heliotrope colouration of the lips and face.' 'Men literally choked to death with pulmonary oedema (swelling), the lungs so swamped with blood, foam and mucous that the faces were grey and the lips purple.' A grey victim might cough up as much as two pints of yellow–green pus per day trying to clear his or her lungs; in so doing, one patient was reported to have ruptured the muscles in his rectum. The purple-black skin was terrifying to doctors, nurses, and family alike. Dr Albert Lamb of New York's Columbia Presbyterian Hospital described the new arrivals as 'blue as huckleberries and spitting blood.'[7] Cyanosis (a bluish discolouration of the skin caused by oxygen deficiency) nearly always meant death within 24–48 hours.[8]

Doctors and scientists from around the world reported a wide range of symptoms. French flu victim Gilberte Boulanger experienced severe nasal haemorrhage – for more than a week, and up to thirty times per day, blood spurted, as if under high pressure, from her nostrils. Other victims, however, complained of a 'burning pain in the diaphragm,' a frontal headache (reminiscent of typhoid fever), and congested and inflamed conjunctivae (the mucous membranes that cover the front of the eyes and line the inside of the eyelids).[7]

The sickness seemed to affect so many organs of the body usually untouched by influenza that Dr Charles Sundell of Britain's Medical Research Council recorded: 'No part of the body is exempt.' Sometimes, for example, the disease was thought to resemble encephalitis, as patients lapsed into coma for three weeks at a time. And sometimes it appeared to mimic nephrosis, as patients, with puffy faces and swollen ankles, passed only ten ounces of blood-streaked urine each day. But the chief of laboratory services at Camp Sherman, Ohio, thought of an attack by chlorine gas – each time a man moved on his pillow, serous fluid poured from his mouth and nose. Still other doctors reported 'silent lungs' – an absence of breath so complete that it was thought that the stethoscope had failed to function.[7]

Perhaps it was 'silent lungs' that sometimes caused a state of 'apparent death.' In Cape Town, South Africa, Kate Le Roux witnessed a wagon loaded with coffins pull away from her friend's house. As she watched, the truck bumped over a pot-hole, and the top-most coffin smashed to the ground, violently releasing its contents. To Kate's horror, the 'corpse' screamed and then scrambled shakily to his hands and knees. In New Mexico, Frank Garundo begged an undertaker to keep his wife Clara's grave open in order that two of his three children, expected to die before the day was over, might be buried with their mother. When baby Helen died, Frank shakily rose from his own sick bed and made the journey to the cemetery. Once there, the grief-stricken man asked that his wife's coffin be opened so that he might take one last look. To his horror, his wife was lying face downwards, with her long black braids twisted in her fingers – testimony to her agony as she tried to escape burial alive.[7]

Just as rumours, stories, and legends abounded of live burials, so, too, did stories of lightning-speed deaths. Charles Lewis of Cape Town boarded a train for his parents' home in Sea Point, only three miles away. The conductor signalled the train's start and immediately died on the platform. Within minutes, a passenger had fallen dead, and the train stopped to unload the body. And then another traveller collapsed. In total, five people were struck down, and five times the train stopped to unload the dead on the pavement for collection by the municipality. And then, with only a quarter of the distance left to travel to Sea Point, the engineer slumped forward and died. Lewis, thrilled to be alive, gladly walked the rest of the way to his destination.[7]

In the United States, a healthy New York woman boarded a subway train for home. When the train pulled into her station forty-five minutes later, she was dead.[10] In Quebec, Canada, a hearse driver infected with Spanish flu toppled from the horse-driven carriage, as if 'struck by lightning.' The man was dead even before he touched the ground. A lone policeman tied a rope to the horse's neck and led the hearse to the cemetery.[7] In Ontario, Canada, two girls sharing a room attended a lecture together one evening when the epidemic was at its height. In the morning, Claire Hunter called to her friend in the same room, 'Vera, I'm going downstairs for breakfast.' There was no response. After breakfast, Claire returned to her room to get her purse and again called to her roommate. No answer. This time, Claire pulled back Vera's sheets. Vera was dead. The doctor said that she had died at about two in the morning.[8]

In many cases, there was no chance for doctors or nurses to intervene. Practitioners were in short supply and overworked, as the war had already siphoned off thousands – 40,000 of 140,000 American doctors had enlisted.[7] When there was a possibility of helping, doctors without therapeutic drugs could turn only to their 'time-honoured cures of rest, liquids and a great deal of hope' to cure very ill patients.[8] Dr Robert Parry of the Middlesex Hospital in London complained that doctors did little more than direct traffic; physicians simply 'guided people to the emergency wards or to the mortuary.'[7]

As thousands of people died, more and more buildings were pressed into use as hospitals. Gymnasiums, chapels, and canteens were all commandeered as temporary hotels for the sick and dying. In Queensland, Australia, the church hall served as the hospital. In Montego Bay, Jamaica, the hospital was the 'Northern News,' and in Enderline, Nebraska, a run-down railway hotel served as the hospital. In St John's, Arizona, the hotel for the sick was the abandoned county jail. Nor was it the only jail to serve; world-famous Sing Sing Prison, 25 miles up the Hudson River from New York City, also did time as a hospital.[7]

In 1918, the medical profession did not know what caused Spanish flu. And because it did not know the cause, it did not know how to prevent the disease. Practitioners rightly assumed that the disease could be spread through the air by coughing or sneezing. Therefore many governments at all levels and on all continents enforced the closure of public areas where people might come into close contact with one another. They closed dance halls, schools, and libraries. Some North American cities shut YMCAs, ice-cream parlours, shoeshine parlours, candy stores, furniture stores, and churches. Some churches did remain open, but their ministers were cautioned to refrain from spitting from the pulpit.[7,8]

Some governments practised quarantine and placarded infected households.[7] In Canada, the Department of Agriculture had administered Quarantine Service from 1867 to 1918, and subsequently the Department of Immigration and Colonization ran it. Unfortunately, Parliament had prorogued on 24 May 1918, and did not resume until 20 February 1919; as a result, there was no central source of advice or control measures.[8] Other governments regulated the wearing of gauze masks. Many masks were decorated: in Rockford, Illinois, they sported a skull and cross-bones.[7] Police in many cities had orders to enforce the wearing of masks and to charge offenders, who were fined.[8] In New York City, huge signs bore the words 'It is Unlawful to Cough and Sneeze' and warned of a $500 fine or a year in jail. Within days, more than 500 New Yorkers had been caught and hauled in front of the courts.[7]

Futile emergency precautions abounded across the continents. In New Zealand, sanitary inspectors, evoking memories of the Black Death, launched a city-wide rat hunt. In Dublin, and in Nottingham, England, mobile water carts poured hundreds of gallons of disinfectant down street gutters. In San Francisco, the law courts were transferred to the open air. In Venice, California, health officers fumigated both animals and performers of the Al. G. Barnes Circus with coal, tar, and formaldehyde. And some townships enforced fumigation of everything from newspapers to tram tickets. Newspapers printed tips on how to keep well: avoid getting chilled; keep hands clean; sleep and work in clean, fresh air; avoid alcoholic stimulants; do not worry; and do not kiss anyone. The U.S. surgeon general recommended avoiding tight clothes, tight shoes, or tight gloves.[7,8,10]

Large numbers of ordinary citizens became afraid to venture outside. Many closed their doors to the outside world in order to stay alive. Instead of visiting friends and family, they communicated via letter. But prior to opening their mail, careful recipients often baked the envelopes to kill any incoming germs.[7,8]

Telephones, still relatively new in 1918, also maintained family ties and friendships. Requests for connecting new lines increased rapidly in Canada. Installers were clearly at risk of exposure to sick families and therefore wore cheesecloth masks soaked in formaldehyde. If the danger seemed especially great, the workmen fastened the phone to a board and pushed it through the house window of a flu-stricken family.[7, 8]

If people did venture outdoors to help friends and relatives, they often risked their own safety and that of their families. Therefore some physicians in Canada and elsewhere recommended one of the many 'vaccinations' against Spanish flu available on the market. All such preventives had their advocates, all had their detractors.[8] Some households, however, had their own methods. Some families wore cotton bags holding camphor or moth balls around their necks to ward off the threat. Others drank violet-leaf tea, inhaled salt water up the nose, or carried hot coals sprinkled with sulphur or brown sugar through the house to avert the danger.[8]

Doctors, in addition to recommending vaccines, made home visits to the sick and dying. They travelled by car, sleigh, horseback, bicycle, and even snowshoe – by whatever means they had available. One medical team left Vancouver Island, British Columbia, in a 12.2-m boat with a large, one-cylinder engine and fought 6.1-m tides on their 136.8-km journey to tend a lumberjack camp.[8]

Poultices of goose-grease, bran, and lard and turpentine and compresses of fir-tree spills, mutton tallow, and mustard were among the concoctions applied to the chests of the sick. Drinks of warm milk, ginger, sugar, pepper, and soda soothed the ill.[7,8] And cough elixirs were administered to strengthen, heal, and make the flu-stricken well. One wholesale drug company that normally sold 6,000 bottles of cough medicine per week now faced a demand of 3,000 per day.[8]

Spanish flu killed an estimated 5 million people in India; in Punjab, the streets were littered with the dead, and trains had to be cleared of dead and dying passengers. In England and Wales, the disease killed an estimated 200,000. Spanish flu wiped out some 550,000 Americans.[7] It killed 19,000 in New York City alone. In Philadelphia, 521 people died in one day, and, at the height of the crisis, 4,500 died in just one week. The local morgue was built for only thirty-six corpses; as a result, several hundred bodies were piled three and four deep. Every room and corridor was packed with the dead – covered with dirty, blood-stained sheets. Before flu disappeared, Philadelphia was forced to open five supplementary morgues to hold the victims.[10]

Canada lost between 30,000 and 50,000. Fourteen thousand perished in Quebec. In Montreal, the demand for transporting coffins was so great that trolley cars had to be converted to hearses which could carry ten coffins at a time. Eight cabinet-makers worked around the clock in Hamilton, Ontario, to keep up with the demand for coffins. Undertakers would take one casket to the cemetery and would hurry back to the church to pick up the next. In Toronto, funerals were allowed on Sunday; white hearses for children became a common sight. So too were sashes on doorways: a white sash for a child; grey for a middle-aged person; and purple for a senior citizen.[8]

Elsewhere in the world, coffins and undertakers were in equally short supply. Many families buried their dead in plain, unvarnished boxes, often fashioned from doors and floorboards. In many countries, however, the dead were interred in cardboard boxes, blankets, or paper shrouds, and piled in mass graves.

In Rio de Janeiro, one householder pleaded with the fire brigade, conscripted as undertakers, to remove his dead brother. They refused, adamant that there was no room on the death cart. However, the desperate brother continued to plead, as the corpse was five days old. The firemen relented; they would take the brother, but in return they would leave a stranger who had died more recently.[7]

In some places, the mortality was much higher than for the world as a whole. For example, in Samoa, 25 per cent of the population died.[7] In Alaska, some villages were wiped out completely, while others lost only their adults; in Nome, 176 of 300 Inuit died of the disease.[10]

The Native population of Okak, Labrador, was equally hard hit: only 59 of 266 people survived. In one home, a man, his wife, and two of their children had died, leaving behind an eight-year-old girl, who survived on her own for five weeks. The Moravian Mission described her ordeal: 'The huskies now began to eat the dead bodies, and the child was a spectator to this horrible incident. So mad the beasts became, upon tasting human flesh, that they attacked the child herself, biting her arm.'[7-8, 12]

The surviving men at Okak dug a pit in the permafrost to bury their dead. It took about two weeks to produce a pit 9.8 m long, 3.1 m wide, and 2.4 m deep. The men dragged the corpses to the excavation. They laid 114 bodies to rest and sprinkled disinfectant over them. Finally the survivors piled rocks on top of the dead to prevent the dogs from tearing at the bodies.[7-8, 12]

At Hebron, Labrador, only 70 people remained of a community of 220. This time there was no pit, and the bodies were simply consigned to the sea. The men quickly cut holes in the ice, weighted the bodies with rocks, and then dropped the corpses through the frozen surface.[7]

During the 1918 pandemic, numerous questions were raised. What caused the 1918 pandemic? Was Spanish flu the same as previous pandemics of influenza? What was the difference between it and the common cold? And what made it so deadly?

Medical practitioners talked of airborne Pfeiffer's bacillus, *Pneumococcus*, *Staphylococcus*, *Streptococcus*, malnourishment, and the crowding together of the world's peoples under conditions of great misery – conditions ideal for an outbreak of infection.[10] Some members of the public, however, explained the pandemic in terms of the weather, cosmic influences, electricity, open windows, closed windows, unclean pyjamas, even sabotage – fish contaminated by the Germans and 'flu germs' released by German U-boats.[13]

Numerous autopsies were performed on the dead, all in the vain hope of locating some identifiable organism – perhaps Pfeiffer's bacillus or *Streptococcus*. Autopsies themselves could be a 'pathological nightmare.' Lungs, saturated with fluid and resembling 'melted red currant jelly,' might be up to six times their normal weight.[7] Sometimes 'bloody fluid oozed out of the lungs sectioned for examination,' and as rigor mortis set in, fluid often poured from a corpse's nose and stained the body wrappings.[9] Other organs, such as the liver, spleen, and kidney, often showed abnormalities, and a few cases even showed swelling of the brain.

If a patient did survive, recovery was often long, slow and painful. One Norwegian nurse, Margit Moller, recalled treating a patient who had lain so long on a pile of newspaper – his only bedding – that flu obituaries for weeks past were imprinted on his buttocks.[7] In Alberta, Canada, Benjamin McKilvington required twenty-one days of recuperation before he could sit up on the edge of his bed. He needed another three weeks to gain enough strength to go outdoors. Still later, he visited the doctor's office, where he was promptly weighed. He weighed only 84 pounds – though wearing two pairs of underwear, two top shirts, a sweater, pants, a heavy overcoat, huge mittens, two pairs of woollen socks, moccasins, and a fur cap – a 'far cry' from his normal 137 pounds.[18]

Throughout the world, those who survived Spanish flu were often left with respiratory weakness. Robert Gain of Quebec City, was hospitalized with flu in December 1918. His wife contracted the disease on New Year's Day, while visiting him at the hospital, and died two weeks later. She left behind five children, aged 18 months to 9 years. Gain's recovery was very slow, and when he returned home in March he lacked the strength to feed himself. He was unable to walk until June.[8]

Whole families disintegrated. Young adults perished and left behind small helpless children, who were often forced into orphanages – 2,000 children in Cape Town and 500 in Stockholm. If young girls were deemed old enough to take over from their dead mothers, they assumed the care of their younger siblings and bore the burdens of adulthood.[7,8]

Throughout the world, losses to businesses were staggering. Merchants suffered because customers were too ill to shop and staff were absent with flu. Theatres, pool halls, and restaurants all lost heavily.[7,8]

But it was the insurance companies that were perhaps the hardest hit. In London, England, the Prudential Assurance Company paid out twice as much in flu claims as it had in war claims. One agent complained: 'It was just as though another large battle was going on in addition to the fighting on all fronts.'[8]

Third Wave

On the tail of this mass destruction came the third and final, less severe wave of Spanish flu. All three waves were over within a period of twelve months in any one country. In some communities, people affected by the first or second wave turned out to be immune to attack in subsequent waves.[10]

In summary, Spanish flu raged in every continent but Antarctica. It infected over half the world's population. Spanish flu killed Prince Erik of Sweden and the dowager queen of the Tongan Islands. Flu also killed General Louis Botha, first premier of the Union of South Africa; Sir Charles Hubert Parry, composer of 'Jerusalem'; and Edmond Rostand, author of *Cyrano de Bergerac*.[7] Survivors included King George V, Crown Prince Max of Baden, the imperial chancellor of Germany, Franklin Delano Roosevelt (U.S. assistant secretary of the navy), and 'Canada's own sweetheart,' actress Mary Pickford.[7]

Deadliest Plague in History

The 1918 influenza is estimated to have killed between 20 million and 40 million people,[14] but not all deaths would have been reported. Many countries had no medical statistics; even in countries that did have figures, physicians were not required to report influenza cases to their boards of health. Not until 1918 was influenza considered sufficiently serious to require recording of cases and deaths. Furthermore, many overworked doctors and nurses may have been too busy and exhausted to keep full reports.[7-10] New estimates suggest that the pandemic may have killed 100 million people.[15] Almost half the deaths occurred among those aged 20–40 years – an age group already devastated by war. 'Spanish influenza killed the prime specimens of those in the prime of life';[10] Spanish flu killed Harry Elionsky, America's strongest swimmer, who had once swum 90 miles non-stop.[7] An acting surgeon general of the U.S. army reported that the infection, like the war, 'kills the young, vigorous, robust adults.'[10] Yet despite its predilection for healthy young people, Spanish flu showed virtually no preference regarding social class or profession.

Has any other plague ever wrought such havoc as Spanish flu? The Black Death, or bubonic plague, which is caused by *Yersinia pestis*, a bacterium carried by fleas that reside on rodents, broke out in 1345, on the steppes of Mongolia. It decimated China's population and rapidly made its way across Asia. From Asia, it marched across Africa and Europe. Daily death rates were staggering: 400 in Avignon, France; 1,500 in Givry, France; 800 in Paris, France; and 500 in Pisa, Italy. In Vienna, the city buried or burned 600 bodies per day.[13] The disease reached Britain in 1348.

Bubonic plague swept from east to west across Europe and then returned from west to east through a new generation of susceptible children. Some people developed pneumonia, which enabled the bacteria to spread by respiratory contagion, killing more than half the population in some cities. London, England, with a pre-plague population of 60,000, was reduced to 35,000; half of Hamburg's population perished, and two-thirds of Bremen's.[13]

In total, the 'Destroying Angel' killed an estimated one-quarter to one-third of the population of Europe (20 million to 30 million people) over more than five years. In the late twentieth century, a new plague – acquired immunodeficiency syndrome (AIDS), caused by the human immunodeficiency virus (HIV) – began spreading rapidly around the planet. The virus spreads through sexual contact with an infected person; through exposure to blood, blood products (for example, through blood transfusion or needle sharing), or tissues of an infected person (for example, through organ transplantation); or by transmission from mother to fetus. As of December 1999, AIDS is thought to have killed 16 million people.

In summary, Spanish flu remains the deadliest disease in recorded history. It killed more people than the bubonic plague of the Middle Ages and more people than AIDS has to date, and, unlike the latter, the 1918 influenza did its killing in only one year.

Possible Connections? Encephalitis Lethargica

In addition to Spanish flu, another worldwide, devastating scourge was raging unabated – encephalitis lethargica – and after a decade of research I still wonder if there are connections between the two. The disease was depicted in the U.S. movie *Awakenings* (1990) based on the pioneering work of Dr Oliver Sacks, as recorded in his book of the same name.[16]

Encephalitis lethargica, known also as von Economo's disease, epidemic encephalitis, and sleeping sickness,[16] appeared suddenly in Austria and France, perhaps as early as 1915, and rapidly picked up momentum. By 1918, it had spread throughout Austria, France, England, Germany, and the United States. By 1919, it had spread over Europe, Canada, Central America, and India. And by 1920, it had diffused throughout the world.[17] The pandemic reached a climax in 1925[18] and rapidly disappeared, as mysteriously as it had appeared, sometime between 1927 and 1930.[19] Its reign of terror had claimed or ravaged the lives of an estimated 5 million people.[16]

The disease began like other types of encephalitis (inflammation of the brain), with fever, headache, stiff neck, and drowsiness.[20] Its symptoms were so varied that few patients ever presented the same picture: 'it was a hydra with a thousand heads.'[16] Some people experienced a dramatic onset, while others were unaware even that they were ill.[19] One child walking home from a concert suddenly developed a headache and then fell into a deep sleep; she died 12 days later without ever waking. 'Roland P.' (not the patient's real name) in *Awakenings* was stricken suddenly at age two-and-a-half by a virulent attack. Overnight, he became intensely drowsy, and he remained so for eighteen weeks. And one 35-year-old woman developed all the signs of post-encephalitic Parkinsonism but could not recall any preceding illness at all.[16] Some victims experienced narcolepsy, stupor, coma, extreme wakefulness, or sleep reversal (they slept through the day and remained awake through the night).[17] Sacks's 'Frances D.' suffered intense insomnia, often resting only two or three hours a night, during her six-month illness. A third of those affected died in the acute stages of sleeping sickness, 'in states of coma so deep as to preclude arousal, or in states of sleeplessness so intense as to preclude sedation.'[16]

Patients who survived an extremely acute attack of somnolence or insomniac illness often 'failed to recover their original aliveness.' If left to themselves, they fell asleep while sitting, standing, walking, or eating. If roused, they woke up quickly and could answer questions or respond to requests. Such patients were like 'extinct volcanoes.' 'They would be conscious and aware – yet not fully awake; they would sit motionless and speechless all day in their chairs, totally lacking energy, impetus, initiative.'[16]

Survivors also suffered from a wide variety of complaints. Parkinsonism (a progressive disease of the nervous system that produces tremor, muscular rigidity, and slowness and imprecision of movements) was perhaps the most common disorder. Many patients became 'living statues – totally motionless for hours, days, weeks, or years.' Other encephalitis disorders included involuntary jerks, spasms, and tics; catatonia; and compulsive actions, such as yawning, coughing, sniffing, gasping, panting, staring, and yelling. Encephalitis lethargica usually spared the higher faculties of 'intelligence, imagination, judgment, and humour.'[16] Patients were then unwilling witnesses to their own horrifying demise.

Child victims suffered less from Parkinsonism than did adults, but they frequently experienced abrupt changes of character. Their sudden disobedient, quarrelsome, and destructive behaviour often led to their expulsion from school. Temper tantrums, stealing, fire-setting, swearing, exhibitionism, and sexual aggression were common. Many children complained that they felt compelled to act badly and as a result were often labelled 'moral imbeciles.'[21]

Some children threatened to kill their friends and families, and a few actually committed murder. One young boy stabbed his mother and threatened 'to cut up' his brother and take a hatchet to his sister. Another youngster, expelled from school for severe behavioural disorders, later broke into uncontrollable fits of rage, attacking and threatening to kill those around him. During his later military service he was frequently punished for his conduct and in fact was sentenced to death (but later reprieved).[22]

Despite the severity of encephalitis lethargica, many patients seemed to make a complete recovery from sleeping sickness and were able to return to their former lives. Their symptom-free recovery period was often followed by post-encephalitic disturbances, with Parkinsonism the most common.[16] Thirty per cent of victims developed Parkinsonian features after three years of recovery, and 50 per cent of victims after five years.[23]

In 1969 Dr Oliver Sacks administered the miracle awakening drug, laevo-dihydroxyphenylalanine, or L-DOPA, to his post-encephalitic patients. In his 1973 book, *Awakenings*, he described his patients' response to the drug: 'For a certain time, in every patient who is given L-DOPA, there is a beautiful, unclouded return to health; but sooner or later, in one way or another, every patient is plunged into problems or troubles. Some patients have quite mild troubles, after months or years of good response; others are uplifted for a matter of days – no more than a moment compared to a life-span – before being cast back into the depths of affliction.'[16]

Sacks awakened 'Mrs. Ida T.,' who, when stricken in Poland by sleeping sickness as a young mother at the age of 20, trebled her weight in just one year. At the same time she had also become increasingly stiff, slow, and violent. Her family shipped her off to the United States for treatment. During her voyage from Poland, she became completely motionless and speechless. On arrival in the United States, she was taken directly to hospital. And for the next 48 years she lay 'rigid, mute, motionless, and glaring.'[16]

In 1969, Sacks administered L-DOPA to Mrs T, 'seal-shaped' and weighing almost 500 pounds. Her body 'suddenly cracked,' and the jubilant woman began walking and talking – 'Wonderful, wonderful! I'm moving inside,' she proclaimed over and over. In 1970, Mrs T. was reunited with her daughter, who had come to the United States in the 1930s. The daughter had never attempted to find her mother because her family had told her that she was dead. It was not an easy reunion, but by 1971 a 'deep mutual relation had been forged.' By 1973, Mrs T. was experiencing some complications – rigidity and stuttering – from the continued use of L-DOPA. However, she was doing very well, considering that she had been catatonic for 48 years.[16]

During the pandemic of encephalitis lethargica, numerous questions arose. Was the disease new, or had it occurred earlier in human history? What was its cause? Was it related to the 1918 influenza?

Baron Constantin von Economo, who first described encephalitis lethargica in 1917 after seeing numerous patients with a strange variety of symptoms at a clinic in Vienna, believed that the disease had probably occurred repeatedly before the Great War. A serious epidemic, described as 'febris comatosa,' had broken out in London, England, between 1673 and 1675. And a severe epidemic, followed by persistent slowness of movement and a lack of initiative in victims, had affected Tubingen, Germany, in 1712 and 1713. Sacks himself has suggested a 2,000-year history.[16] Von Economo had warned that the causative agent 'was not extinct but only in a dormant or non-virulent form from which it would invariably re-emerge as it has done innumerable times since the dawn of recorded time.'[23]

He was right. Occasional cases have been reported since the 1950s.[24–8] Their significance is, however, not clear, and it is not known if they are caused by the same pathogen. No causative agent was identified during the pandemic, but since its clinical and pathological features were typical of a viral infection, medical practitioners immediately questioned whether sleeping sickness was related to Spanish flu.

The recently examined brains of six people who died from encephalitis lethargica have shown antigens for the influenza A viral strains WSN and NWS, indicating exposure to these particular strains.[23]

There is some good circumstantial evidence linking the Spanish flu and sleeping sickness.[29] Both pandemics were globally distributed and were closely related in time. Local, regional, and national epidemics of Spanish flu invariably preceded 'similar-sized' outbreaks of encephalitis lethargica.[30] Both diseases showed a preference for young, healthy people. Deaths were greatest in the 20–40-year age groups for Spanish flu and in the 20s–50s for sleeping sickness.[23] A large number of victims of encephalitis lethargica had had influenza in 1918. And finally, past pandemics of encephalitis have been recorded in close association with other influenza epidemics; for example, the great influenza epidemic of 1889–90 preceded the notorious 'nona' – a severe somnolent illness that was followed by Parkinsonism in almost all survivors.[30]

Deniers of links between the two diseases would, however, probably plead that von Economo himself found no relationship. In 1931, he wrote, 'The first cases (of encephalitis lethargica) occurred as early as 1915 and settle once and for all the fact that encephalitis appeared certainly two and possibly three years before the first appearance of the influenza epidemic.'[23] Furthermore, influenza was highly communicable from person to person, whereas encephalitis was remarkably non-communicable. Nor did all cases of encephalitis lethargica have a history of preceding influenza infection. Finally, not all influenza epidemics are associated with epidemic encephalitis.[30] Despite the arguments, the balance of circumstantial evidence suggests that the two diseases may be related.

Summary

The second and third decades of the twentieth century experienced two great plagues, which remain mysteries even today: Spanish flu, the deadliest disease in recorded history, and encephalitis lethargica.

The two claimed the lives of millions worldwide, and both changed families and the course of history. Following the two crises, scientists doggedly studied the pandemics and tracked their paths of destruction. More important, they continued to search for causes in hope of preparing for the next influenza pandemic – perhaps one that could prove as lethal as that of 1918 – and the next outbreak of sleeping sickness.

Part One

An Evolving Team

2   The Quest

1992–1994

The cause of the great influenza pandemic had to be found. The plea was heard in the streets and from labs and governments around the world in 1918. Monkeys, rabbits, and human volunteers were inoculated with sputum and juices from the lungs of the dead in the hopes of showing that something – bacteria or viruses – was being passed between patients. Unfortunately, no illness was produced because scientists failed to drop the infected materials into the nasal passages – the route by which infection was transmitted.

Fifteen years after the 'Spanish Lady' visited, scientists Christopher Andrews and Wilson Smith of the National Institute for Medical Research (NIMR) at Mill Hill in London, England, isolated the first human influenza virus. They carefully dropped throat washings from human influenza victims for the first time into the noses of ferrets. The transmissibility of the virus was later discovered when a sick ferret sneezed in a scientist's face, and the man became ill a few days later.[1]

Much has been learned over the past six decades about influenza – from the structure of the virus to control methods for infections.

The Virus

Influenza is a unique respiratory viral disease infecting the whole respiratory tract – namely, the nose, sinuses, the throat, lungs, and even the middle ear. The disease spreads from person to person by airborne droplets produced when an infected individual coughs or sneezes. Acute symptoms of influenza, including fever, headache, shivering, muscle pain, cough, and pneumonia, are the result of the virus repli-

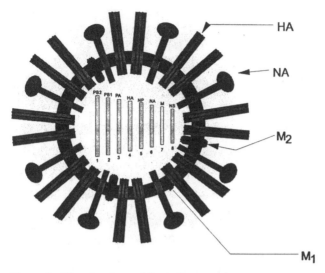

Figure 1   The structure of the influenza virus.

cating in the respiratory tract, where infected cells die and slough off.[2]

The influenza virus exists in three forms – called A, B, and C – but only A and B cause significant disease in humans. Despite the virus's three forms, all influenza viruses look similar. Influenza viruses are roughly spherical particles, 80–120 nanometres (nm) in diameter, containing a nucleoprotein core of RNA and a lipid envelope from which two distinct forms of glycoprotein project – the rod-shaped haemagglutinin (H) and the mushroom-shaped neuraminidase (N) (Figure 1). A third protein structure, called the matrix (M1) protein layer, lines the surface of the virus and contains M2 molecules.[3]

Haemagglutinin is highly variable; neuraminidase is more constant. The variation that occurs in H and N surface antigens has allowed influenza viruses to be classified into three main antigenic haemagglutinin subtypes (H1, H2, and H3) and two neuraminidase subtypes (N1 and N2). The three principal strains of influenza that affect humans are H1N1, H2N2, and H3N2.[2] Strain H5N1, which originated in 1997 in chickens in Hong Kong, has been shown to be particularly virulent; authorities decided to kill every chicken (many millions) in Hong Kong to prevent the deadly avian flu from spreading.[3]

Individual Type A influenza strains are also designated by origin, isolate number, year of isolation, and subtype; for example, one strain is referred to as Influenza A/Hong Kong/3/79 H3N2 – or Hong Kong flu.[3]

There is no effective cure that works against all influenza viruses. Current prevention takes place by annual vaccination, particularly for high-risk groups such as those with respiratory disease, heart disease, renal trouble, and diabetes.[3]

Because the virus is able to change surface antigens, each year the influenza virus is a little different. However, sometimes the changes are major, often with an entire viral gene segment being replaced by one from an animal influenza virus, and it is these major changes that lead to pandemics. Because the virus changes, so too does the vaccine. Therefore the World Health Organization (WHO), which involves 100 national centres in its influenza-surveillance program, reviews the make-up of the vaccine each year. The WHO then makes recommendations regarding the strains of influenza virus that it considers will be most prevalent in the coming flu season. Vaccines are then produced to combat those strains.[3]

Vaccination is given by intra-muscular injection, 6–8 weeks before the influenza season. In general, most studies suggest that vaccines reduce the frequency of severe illness 'but do less to reduce the overall frequency of infection.' The closer the vaccine is in structure to the antigenic composition of the circulating strain of virus, the more effective it is. Vaccine efficacy varies greatly from about 20 per cent to as high as 90 per cent, depending on patient group. Protection rates of 70 per cent to 90 per cent can be achieved in healthy young adults when vaccine and epidemic strains match closely.[3]

Anti-viral drugs, such as amantadine and rimantidine, can attenuate influenza infection, but they have an effect on only influenza A and quickly lead to development of resistance. Moreover, their side effects include anxiety, concentration problems, nausea, headache, dizziness, insomnia, and, rarely, delirium, behavioural changes, and hallucination.[3]

Finally, over-the-counter medication, such as Aspirin, Tylenol, and ibuprofen, with their analgesic and fever-reducing properties, has been used to reduce some of the discomfort caused by the influenza infection. A plethora of drugs is also available to help ease sore throats, reduce coughing, unblock sinuses, and so on. Unfortunately, none of these drugs has any effect on the underlying influenza infection.[3]

But despite the advances in identification of the virus and prevention of infection, there is a need for new options for the control of influenza, especially lethal varieties such as Spanish flu. The much-publicized outbreak of 'chicken flu' in Hong Kong in 1997 highlighted the on-going threat of a pandemic.[3]

Deadly flus seem to occur three times a century, and so we are perhaps due for a killer flu. Could Spanish flu reappear in the future? The answer – maybe. And if it should, the world must be prepared.

Two 1950s Expeditions

In the 1950s, two American-led teams planned to be ready for such an eventuality – they would exhume frozen victims of the Spanish flu in the hopes of identifying the virus that killed them. In 1951, a team from the University of Iowa led by Dr Albert McKee and his graduate student Johan Hultin descended on Teller Mission on Alaska's Seward Peninsula to unearth the bodies of Inuit victims of the Spanish flu. In 1918, all but eight of the 115 Inuit at the Mission died of the disease. The deaths had occurred so quickly, and there were so many bodies, that the Mission called in the U.S. army. The troops used a steam generator to thaw the permafrost before burying the bodies in a common grave.[4] In 1951, after receiving the necessary permissions – from the governor, the state health commissioner, and the chief of the village – members of the University of Iowa team excavated at one end of the mass grave. They took small samples of lung from four perfectly preserved, 'but a little dried out,' victims, flew the samples back to the continental United States, and in the privacy of their lab tried unsuccessfully to recover the world's most frightening disease agent.[5] They left little information behind.

Also in 1951, the U.S. army's Project George undertook a similar exercise without, according to Dr Albert McKee, the necessary permissions. The details of the project remain classified.[5,6] According to Emily Court, reference librarian for the Armed Forces Medical Library, *The Armed Forces Epidemiological Board: The History of the Commissions* makes no mention of the army's attempt to recover the live virus from Alaskan bodies.[6] Court also requested in 1998, on my behalf, that the offices of the Epidemiological Board attempt to locate information on Project George. She wrote back to me: 'We have ... checked a database of documents; we weren't able to locate anything ... Two large folders which covered the Commission on Influenza from approximately 1942 through February, 1955 ... I went through every page, and there was nothing about Project George.'[6] She faxed me a ProMed communication from Hal Houser written in June 1996. He re-read the report and wrote that there was 'no mention of or allusion to the events in Alaska. This doesn't mean that they didn't happen, or ... neglected to include them. It is more likely that the record has been lost, destroyed or is otherwise undiscoverable.'[5–10]

Continuing the Quest: Looking for Information, Samples, and Victims

In the early 1990s, seventy-five years after the initial outbreaks, the scientific world still knew nothing about the identity of the causal agents of Spanish flu and encephalitis lethargica. They had become two of the world and history's greatest medical mysteries.

In 1992, reading about flu's gruesome effects and the experts' alarming predictions made me want to investgate both diseases. However, I am not a virologist or a neuropathologist. I am a geographer. I have taught meteorology, climatology, climate change, and medical geography. In 1992, I knew nothing about influenza or sleeping sickness: strike one. I was young and had virtually no track record: strike two. I am a woman: strike three. Although I did not know it, I was to find that there are barriers for women in science, particularly for relatively young women. Nevertheless, I felt driven to solve the unanswered puzzles. This is the story of the voyage that followed.

The quest began with my searching for all available information on influenza and sleeping sickness. Medline – a computer search tool for the health sciences – listed thousands of articles on influenza but only a few on encephalitis lethargica, as that disease largely disappeared by the late 1920s, except for a few suspected, isolated cases. I spent weeks at the computer reading abstract after abstract – sometimes hundreds in one day – and then searched the stacked library shelves at the University of Toronto for each important article.

This was the beginning of my six-month crash course in virology. I diligently read each article, book, monograph, and commissioned report listed on Medline, afraid to miss any scrap of potentially valuable information. I made detailed notes on the aetiology, epidemiology, clinical features, diagnosis, treatment, prevention, and control of influenza and encephalitis lethargica. I memorized the dates and details of the outbreaks, the epidemics, and the influenza pandemics of the last five centuries, and I studied the language of a new science.

· When I completed my review of the current literature, I descended into the lower levels of the University of Toronto's Gerstein Medical Library to examine fading articles and books from the early decades of the twentieth century. It was difficult poring over case histories. But after six months of intensive research, I felt ready to approach the experts.

I required pathological samples of lung and brain tissue from 1918 and from the 1920s. I phoned leading virologists to ask if tissues existed from victims of either Spanish influenza or encephalitis lethargica. I then asked leading neuropathologists for samples from victims of sleeping sickness. The experts all informed me that no samples existed; nevertheless, archival samples would surface later.

I then began tracking down the team members of the University of Iowa and the U.S. army expeditions. Did samples remain from their scientific studies? The answer was always 'no.' However, Dr Albert McKee, leader of the university expedition, suggested that I phone the universities where he had worked since 1951 to inquire if samples were stored in some back corner of a freezer. I did so. The precious samples had long since disappeared.

Six months of reading, and I was stuck. I decided to search for bodies, rather than for archival samples. My geography training came in handy – I thought of permafrost. I hoped, just as the U.S. army and the university team had, that frozen ground would have preserved the bodies along with whatever bug had killed the victims.

Before beginning my search for victims, I made one last round of calls to the experts, such as Dr Daniel Perl, a neuropathologist at Mount Sinai Hospital in New York City, and Dr Susan Daniel, a neuropathologist at the United Kingdom's Parkinson Disease Society Brain Tissue Bank in London, England. I also spoke with Dr Charles Smith, a pathologist, and Dr Peter Lewin, a paediatrician and medical archaeologist, both from the world-famous Hospital for Sick Children in Toronto. I briefly explained my idea and asked if they might be interested in working with me. The answer was a resounding 'yes.' If I found victims, I was to call them.

I needed to find victims. I thought first of Alaska. After all, there had been two previous searches there, the population had been decimated by influenza, and there were broad expanses of permafrost. But had encephalitis lethargica ever reached Alaska? To answer this question I required death certificates with 'cause of death' from the state.

I contacted Alaska's Bureau of Vital Statistics. Photocopies of death certificates from 1918 and 1924 would cost over $2,000. Death certificates from 1918 would no doubt include deaths from Spanish flu, and certificates from 1924 might record victims of sleeping sickness, which peaked in 1925. I needed a grant. The University of Windsor, where I was an assistant professor of geography, provided the necessary money, and the bureau issued the documents.

An examination of the 1918 records revealed, as I expected, endless deaths of influenza victims. Unfortunately, key information was often missing. Frequently no doctor or nurse visited the dying or the dead. There were often no burial data: no place of death or place of interment. There was frequently no personal information: no name, no age, no details about the life so ruthlessly snatched away. Yet despite the scanty information, I was able to compile a short list of Spanish flu victims with known cause of death (that is, the victims had been seen by a medical practitioner) and recorded place of interment.

My search of 1924 certificates revealed no victims of sleeping sickness. The deaths, however, clearly reflected the frontier nature of the territory, with accidents claiming almost 20 per cent of all male victims for the year. Of the accidental deaths, drowning was the most frequent cause, followed by freezing, falls, and shootings.

Detailed reviews of the medical and historical literature also failed to turn up information regarding sleeping sickness in Alaska. My last chance: call the state's medical practitioners. Did they know of sleeping sickness in the state? Had they treated post-encephalitic victims? The answer was 'no' to both questions.

However, there were records of flu victims. I had to compare their places of interment with a detailed permafrost map to determine if any had been buried in frozen ground. I phoned the permafrost experts at the American Geological Survey and asked for detailed maps of the location and extent of permafrost in Alaska. I learned that no such maps existed.[11] A detailed map was not produced until 1997,[12] four years after my request. After six months of examining death certificates, I found my research blocked again.

There was no point in considering Iceland, which had been decimated by the influenza pandemic. Iceland's geothermal energy would never allow for biological preservation.[13]

My next thoughts were of Russia, which, like Alaska and Iceland, had been devastated by Spanish influenza. I wrote to leading medical authorities informing them of my interest and got no response to any of my requests. However, I have since learned (1996) from the U.S. Army Medical Research Institute of Infectious Diseases (USAMRIID) in Frederick, Maryland, and from the Centers for Disease Control (CDC) and Prevention in Atlanta, Georgia, that Russian scientists are communicating with their American counterparts regarding the possibility of unearthing flu victims in order to find the causal agent of the 1918 pandemic.

After two years of searching, I still had nothing. I needed a break. And the break did come – from Scotland. My dear friend Dr Andrew Kerr called from the University of Edinburgh's Geography Department. The building housing the department had previously served as the Royal Infirmary of Edinburgh, where Charles Darwin had once laboured in the upstairs laboratories.

Andy told me about his recent trip across a glacier in Spitsbergen; he also mentioned rifles, flares, dried foods, and rigorous disposal methods for human waste. I listened with interest. And then he mentioned permafrost.

Permafrost! I became excited. I knew that flu had hit Norway. In fact, more than 7,300 people had died there of Spanish flu, and more than 370,000 were registered as having had the disease. I realized that if people had travelled from Norway to Svalbard, they might have carried influenza with them. And if flu had raged, sleeping sickness perhaps followed.

I wrote immediately to the Norsk Polarinstitutt (Norse Polar Institute) in Longyearbyen, Svalbard, and briefly described my research interests.

Svalbard

I knew very little of the environs or history of Spitsbergen and the archipelago, Svalbard. While I waited for a response to my letter to Longyearbyen, I immersed myself in the history and geography of the region. Svalbard, its wonderful people, and seven of its dead were to become, and still are, the focus of my life and of our project.

History

Stone-age tools suggest that one or more cultures may have existed in Svalbard about 3000 BC. A mythical Svalbard, mentioned in the Norse sagas of 1194, may indicate that the group of islands was discovered in

1194. And dated timber remains of Pomor hunting stations may imply that Russian hunters visited in the mid-sixteenth century.[14]

On 17 June 1596, the Dutch mariner Willem Barentsz wrote, 'It was calm to noon but when we reached the 80th degree and 10 minutes we weighed ... to go around the ice, passed at 6 leagues ... Went even a quarter mile further with wind SE, went SSW 4 leagues. Then we saw land and went again WSW, ... the land is high and all covered by snow.' Barentsz's detailed account and later map 'leave no doubt' that the land that he discovered was Svalbard, or, more precisely, northwestern Spitsbergen. Navigator Henry Hudson in 1607 reported an abundance of sea mammals in the fjords. A massive assault on the whales followed, as Europeans demanded the huge cetaceans' oil for lamp fuel, lubricating oil, and soap, and baleen for clothing.[14]

In the seventeenth century, the 'Spitsbergen Fishery' consisted of some 1,650 whaling ships carrying double crews of 70–80 men. One crew would helm the ship and hunt the 20-m, 100-tonne Greenland whales, while the other chopped and boiled blubber at land stations such as the infamous 'Smeerenburg,' or 'Blubber town.'[14,15] The tonnage varied from one season to another. In 1722, Dutch whalers alone caught 1,100 whales, which yielded some 58,000 quartels ('tuns of 233 litres') of train-oil and nearly 500 tons of whalebone. In the eighteenth and nineteenth centuries, trapping and hunting of birds, reindeer, polar fox, and polar bear became popular among Russian and Norwegian trappers, who occupied winter cabins scattered along Svalbard's coast. One trapper is believed to have spent an incredible thirty-nine winters there.[14]

Svalbard's present wave of coal-mining began in 1899, the year that the archipelago's first shipment of coal reached mainland Norway. Within a few years, many mines opened. The American capitalist John Monroe Longyear, and Frederick Ayer established the Arctic Coal Company (ACC) in 1904. From 1906–1916, ACC operated Mine 1A, whose entrance still stands on the mountainside above the present-day cemetery.[14,15]

The work beneath the ground was both arduous and dangerous. At ACC, the workers went on strike in 1906, 1910, and 1912 to protest poor working and housing conditions. The men worked eight hours underground in a ten-hour day. In 1920, twenty-six miners were killed by a coal-dust explosion and fire in Mine 1A. Off-duty miners lived in barracks housing fifty men each. Home comforts were minimal; miners were required to remove the day's coal dust by means of melted snow in tin basins.[14]

A small town rapidly developed around ACC's mine and was named Longyear City – the present Longyearbyen. By 1919, the population had grown to 230, including 37 women and children. Two years later, the 350 residents had such amenities as church, cinema, hospital, mess hall, and sauna. Coal companies gradually became concentrated into a few major mines, including Store Norske Spitsbergen Kulkompani (SNSK), the former ACC.[14] Since 1916, SNSK has developed six mines in the vicinity of Longyearbyen; two are still in production today.[15]

Miners of many nationalities – British, Dutch, German, Norwegian, Russian, and Swedish – fought for mining rights in the archipelago. Ownership of Svalbard was unresolved until the Svalbard Treaty of 1920 awarded Norway sovereignty and granted mineral rights on an equal basis to all the signatories. The treaty forbade the islands to be used for 'warlike purposes.' Norway formally integrated Svalbard on 14 August 1925.[14]

Svalbard was evacuated in August and September 1941. Coal and oil stores were set on fire, and equipment was made inoperable, to prevent the Germans from using the valuable supplies. The Germans soon invaded Svalbard and established a small garrison in Longyearbyen with a temporary airfield and a meteorological station.[14]

A small expeditionary force under Einar Sverdrup, director of SNSK, was sent to Barentsburg in May 1942 because weather observations were important to the Allies and because Sverdrup wanted to maintain the coal mines. The expedition's two small ships were spotted and attacked by German aircraft. The survivors set up a garrison at Barentsburg.[14]

The Germans regularly made reconnaissance flights over Svalbard, or visited the fjords with submarines. And in September 1943 the infamous *Tirpitz*, sister ship of the *Bismarck*, with *Scharnhorst* and nine destroyers attacked and almost completely destroyed Barentsburg, Grumant, and Longyearbyen. The Nazis apparently believed the Allied forces in Svalbard to be considerably greater in number than the 152 soldiers actually present.[14]

Rebuilding of Longyearbyen began in 1945, and soon coal production from the Norwegian mines reached pre-war levels. In 1948, 420,000 tons was shipped to mainland Norway. Since the Second World War, coal production has been unprofitable. Norwegian and foreign oil companies have prospected unsuccessfully for oil and gas since the 1960s. Trapping too has decreased dramatically, especially after 1972, when the government moved to protect the polar bear.[14]

Svalbard continued to grow, especially with the opening of the airport in 1975. Today people in Spitsbergen's Norwegian settlements enjoy television and telephone, regular air communication with the mainland, and high net incomes.[14]

Settlements

Svalbard is home to only 4,500 people, who live in either Norwegian or Russian communities. The majority live on Spitsbergen, and Longyearbyen, nestled within Longyeardalen (Longyear Valley), is the main Norwegian centre. Most of the community's 1,100 inhabitants work either for SNSK, responsible for Norwegian coal-mining activities in Longyearbyen and Sveagruva, or for the governor of Svalbard (Sysselmannen Pa Svalbard).[15–17] SNSK owns and operates family apartments spread over 2–3 km along the floor of Longyeardalen. The church, school, and hospital are run by the Norwegian government.[18]

The community boasts an education system covering the years from kindergarten to university and activities ranging from airplane and helicopter rides to scuba diving and wind surfing – all just 1,300 km from the North Pole. Other forms of recreation include biking, boating, dog-sled rides, fossil hunting, hiking, mine visits, parachuting, 'scooter' or snowmobile rides, and skiing.[16]

Other communities on Spitsbergen include Barentsburg, a Russian town of 1,400 people, and Pyramiden, with 1,000 residents.[18] Ny-Alesund was the most northern coal mine and settlement in the world at 79°N; today it is the primary centre of scientific research in Svalbard.[16]

Geography

'Svalbard' is an Old Norwegian name meaning 'cold coast' and aptly describes the islands, rocks, and skerries lying 1,000 km north of the Norwegian mainland and only 500 km from the northeastern tip of Greenland.[18] Svalbard, a mere speck on a map of the world, is in reality a large archipelago of 62,400 km^2, lying between latitude 74° and 81°N and longitude 10° and 35°E. The group of islands is roughly one-fifth

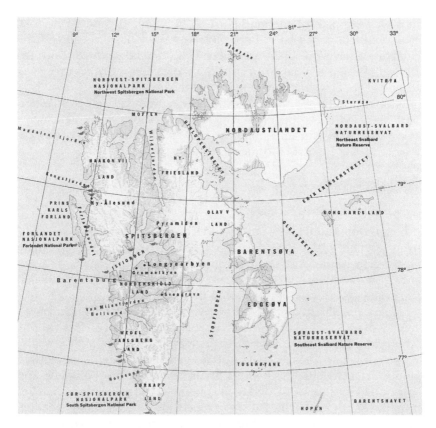

Figure 2   Svalbard Archipelago.

the extent of Norway, or approximately the size of Canada's Nova Scotia (Figure 2).[18] Spitsbergen, the largest island, covers 39,000 km^2. Penetrating deep into the largest islands are long fjords, such as Isfjorden, which cuts far into the interior of Spitsbergen.[18]

The archipelago's rocky underpinning, dating from the Precambrian to the present, includes deposits with coal and, potentially, oil, natural gas, and gypsum.[16] The varied geology determines the landscape: in northernmost areas of Spitsbergen, granites and gneiss give the mountains their characteristic rounded shape; along its west coast heavily folded and metamorphic rock strata form magnificent, jagged mountains, and peaks that exceed 1,700 m in height.[18]

Glaciers cover two-thirds of Svalbard. Ice caps are typical of the east, while valley glaciers and mountain ice-fields predominate in the west. Permafrost extends to a remarkable depth of about 500 m in some places but to only 100 m along the coast.[18] The topmost, active layer of the permafrost (1.0–1.5 m in depth) thaws for a brief period each summer.[19]

Svalbard, despite its location north of the Arctic Circle, enjoys a rather balmy mean annual temperature of –4.8°C.[16,17] The Gulf Stream, or North Atlantic Drift, carries vast quantities of warm, tropical water northwards and heats the archipelago.[20] As a result, mean monthly temperatures range from –16.0°C for the winter months to 6.0°C for the summer months. Only during June, July, and August do temperatures remain reliably above freezing.[15]

Svalbard receives a meagre average annual precipitation of about 200 mm.[15] In lower latitudes, such minimal precipitation would constitute a desert climate, but since evaporation rates are very low and moisture remains adequate, a tundra climate results in cold polar regions.[20]

Midnight sun is visible from mid-April until mid-August, and polar night, the period of total darkness, lasts from roughly mid-October to mid-February.[16] After darkness has fallen, an eerie, but dazzling light show – the northern lights, or aurora borealis – often appears in the sky. The light dances across the heavens in a yellow–green arc much wider than a rainbow, or the light decorates the sky as flickering draperies of blue, green, and purple.[20] The Sami, Norway's aboriginal people, believe that there is a power in the aurora borealis that commands respect – a 'power stronger than the strength of man.'[21] Scientists, too, appreciate the great power, for, at its peak, an auroral display can produce more than a billion watts of power.[20]

Flora and Fauna

More than half of Svalbard consists of protected areas, such as national parks, nature and plant reserves, and bird sanctuaries.[22,23] The region's 165 species of vegetation cover only 10 per cent of the land mass; the most fertile areas are served by the fjords of the west and north. Dwarf birches are the only trees, as the vegetation is limited by thin soils, low temperatures, little rainfall, and a short growing season.[22]

Arctic fox, Svalbard reindeer, and polar bear, or 'isbjorn' (ice bear), roam freely across the archipelago.[14] The polar bear, which can weigh as much as 700 kilos, is one of the world's largest predators.[23] Capable of charging across the frozen tundra at 50 km per hour, the adult polar bear is a formidable predator of Svalbard's whales, walruses, seals, and even humans.[22] But it most commonly eats ringed seals, which make dens in the snow on the frozen sea.[23] 'When a bear smells a seal through the snow, it ... plunges into the den nose first, grabbing the seal's head in its jaws and crushing its skull.' It has a different way of attacking seals that have just poked their noses through an icy blowhole for a breath of air. 'They hit the ice hard ... The force of the ice crushes the seal's skull.' The bear then locks the seal or 400-kg walrus in its jaws and pulls the animal through.[24] It can attack humans suddenly, quickly, and without warning. The majestic ice bear is, however, protected by law and 'must in no way be disturbed or pursued.'[22]

Seven on Spitsbergen

I had spent weeks of immersion in 'everything Svalbard' when a letter arrived, postmarked 'Norway.' It was a response to my request for information from the Norse Polar Institute in Longyearbyen. I eagerly tore into the envelope and quickly skimmed the much-anticipated letter. Yes, yes, thank you for your request. Yes, interesting. Difficult task ahead. Apparently few records were available from 1918. There were no government records, since Svalbard did not officially become part of Norway until 1925. No medical records were available, because the hospital had been destroyed during the Second World War. No church records existed, since the first minister did not journey to Longyearbyen until 1920. I continued to skim the letter. Diaries existed – 'Sigurd Vestbyes Dagboker' – kept by SNSK.

I did not finish the letter but instead phoned SNSK. 'The director, please.' The line crackled. 'My name is Dr Duncan. I am calling from Canada. I am looking for diaries kept by the coal company in 1918 and 1924.'

A long pause. I waited with bated breath. And then the answer, 'We no longer have the diaries; they are gone.' Gone. How could they be gone?

I asked timidly if copies existed. I must have sounded anxious. 'Yes, yes,' he laughed. 'The school master and curator of the museum [one person] has them.' I was excited again and eventually tracked down Mr Mork, the teacher, who had the diaries and would be pleased to translate them for me.

Several weeks later, I received Mork's translation of the 1918 and 1921 diaries. The 1918 document recorded the unleashing of Spanish flu in

Spitsbergen. There was no record of sleeping sickness. I excitedly read the faded photocopy of one page in history. 'July 27th, 12 persons sick. July 28th, 14 more persons sick. 29th. 50 men to the Doctor. 30th. Spanish flu has come! Extra medicine from Norway! ... July 31st. 25 men at work. Rest of men sick with Spanish flu. August 7th. Sick men from Green Harbour near Barentsburg had to stay on board ship. August 8th. First person died. August 18th. One new patient from Kapp Thorsden. Isolation is no help. 20th. Three died.'[25]

Next: 'This season's last ship. 7 men died and were buried on October 27th 1918 in the churchyard at Longyearbyen.'[25] The seven miners sailed on the last ship of the season, *Forsete*, to work in Svalbard's coal mines. The ship left Tromso on 21 September 1918 for Longyear City with sixty-nine healthy, young people. All of them fell ill during the two-day crossing, but none of the crew succumbed to Spanish flu, as they had all been sick with flu earlier that summer. Some passengers were so ill that they were taken straight to the hospital (which had a licensed physician); others, however, were boarded in the miners' barracks. The quarters were extremely cramped, with three bunks piled one on top of another. As a result, Spanish flu once again swept through the Arctic community.[26]

On 29 September, *Forsete* returned to Norway with twenty-nine convalescents on board. Subsequently, between 1 and 7 October, seven patients died. Later the sea froze, and further communication by sea became impossible until May 1919.[26]

The seven miners who would become the focal point of my planned project died during the first week of October, during the deadly autumn wave of the Spanish flu pandemic; the summer outbreak in Spitsbergen may have given the population immunity, and may explain why only incoming miners died in the autumn. The seven miners were between 19 and 28 years of age – the range typical of victims of Spanish flu throughout the world.

At last, after two years of searching, I had found victims. My excitement was, however, tempered by the fact that Spanish flu was no longer an anonymous scientific puzzle, a great faceless mystery. I wondered who the young men were and whether they had been excited or fearful on journeying to a new land. Were they travelling to Spitsbergen to start a new life? Did they have dreams of a new beginning? Whom did they leave behind?

And I thought about their fears – of a hostile environment, of a dark, cold mine, of perhaps never seeing family again, and of dying. The 'Spanish Lady' was aboard their ship. Passengers became sick; so did the young men. Everyone aboard the ship would have had some experience with the deadly flu; it was the autumn, and the disease had been raging since the spring. Were the young men afraid? Did they know that they were dying? Did they know that they would never return to their homeland and would forever lie on a barren slope overlooking Longyearbyen?

Finding the sad records of the seven young miners was only the first step in a long voyage. There would be many steps to follow. It was first necessary to determine if the miners' graves were marked and if the graves had been disturbed. If there were no markers, the project would have been virtually impossible. If the bodies had been moved, or if they had been dug up by animals, there could be no project. I wrote to Per Arne Engdal, the pastor of Svalbard Kirke, who informed me that the graves were marked by white crosses and that they had not been disturbed. The news was encouraging.

The next step was to determine the burial customs of Spitsbergen in 1918. I contacted archaeologists, historians, the Lutheran church, Norwegian funeral directors, and government authorities. I was informed that bodies without embalming fluid were placed in simple, wooden coffins and buried. This was promising information; if cremations had been undertaken, there could be no project. The fact that embalming fluid was not used is important because a preserving agent could have altered the structure of the influenza virus.

The archaeologists, historians, and others agreed that the miners would probably have been interred at a depth of 2 m, according to Norway's law in 1918. A deep burial would assure cold ground temperatures and a good chance of the bodies being preserved.

But Spitsbergen was no man's land in 1918. It had no government and no church; the only rules were those of the coal companies. Therefore it was impossible to know at what depth the young men were interred. But there was some good evidence to suggest that the young men were buried rather deep. First, the men died in October, the time of the greatest melting of the permafrost and thus the time of easiest digging. The bodies had not floated to the surface of the ground (as they had in other parts of Svalbard), which suggested that they were buried deeply in the permafrost. Mining-town residents knew how to dig in the permafrost and could therefore dig deeply into the ground. And finally, the inhabitants of Longyearbyen, who already knew Spanish flu and were likely very afraid of it, would have wanted to bury the men deeply to prevent their resurfacing in the future.

My next question was whether ground temperatures had been cold enough to allow the preservation of biological material over the last eighty years. I contacted Alan Heginbottom of the Geological Survey of Canada, a permafrost specialist, to determine the ground temperatures over the last many decades for the depths at which the miners were assumed to be buried.

Alan determined that at a depth of 1.0–1.5m, the ground temperatures would have ranged between –10.0 and –4.0°C over the last seventy-seven years. These temperatures are considerably colder than those in a standard morgue (4°C) and would thus allow preservation of the body and, perhaps, of viral material.

After searching for 2½ years, I had put together an ideal case. I had found the resting places of seven miners who had died of Spanish influenza. Their graves were marked and had been undisturbed for almost eight decades. The burial practices of the time were appropriate to allow sampling of the miners' tissues. And the depth of the burials and the temperatures at those depths were also suitable for sampling.

I should have been elated. But I was finding my planned project – to take small samples of tissue from the seven miners in order to characterize the Spanish flu virus – extremely difficult. I believe that a person's final resting place is sacred and that a body should not be disturbed during its long rest.

Should I proceed with the exhumations or not? This was the first of many ethical decisions to make along the way. On the one hand, there was a chance that the results of the planned project could improve human health. Identifying the causal agent of Spanish flu might allow scientists to explain why it had killed so many and why it had disappeared so quickly. Describing the causal agent might allow scientists to improve current influenza vaccines and test present anti–viral drugs against the deadly flu. On the other hand, the project went against my beliefs about the inviolability of graves.

Finally, my father spoke; he said that if his body held the answers to a deadly disease, he hoped that someone would come along and unravel those secrets. It was my father's words that allowed me to take the next step – to put together a research team to collaborate with me.

3 Beneath the Crosses

1994–May 1996

A Multinational Team

To build a research team, I assumed, I would choose leading scientists from around the world, and we would all work together to solve the mysteries of Spanish flu and encephalitis lethargica. In 1994, I believed that this could happen. But I knew that I would have an uphill struggle. Science, like other professions, includes a unique blend of personalities, egos, and politics. The initial team, however, included excellent people – three Canadians, three Americans from CDC, and experts (American, British, Canadian) in encephalitis lethargica. Dr Charles Smith, Dr Peter Lewin, and Mr Alan Heginbottom – all Canadians – saw the project through to fruition.

Charles Smith is a paediatric forensic pathologist at Toronto's Hospital for Sick Children ('Sick Kids') and an associate professor in the Faculty of Medicine at the University of Toronto. I met him in 1993 to discuss the epidemiology of sudden infant death syndrome (SIDS) for another project on which I was working. We met at Ontario's Paediatric Forensic Pathology Unit, which performs post-mortem examinations of children who have died suddenly or under suspicious circumstances. On the elevator ride up to the unmarked pathology floor, I wondered what kind of person chooses to be a pathologist and what qualities such a specialist requires. My first thoughts: such an individual would be detached, cool, and unemotional, particularly if he works with the bodies of children and daily witnesses trauma, abuse, and neglect of young people. However, I was greeted by a warm, smiling, tall, blond man, sporting a Bugs Bunny tie, who quickly ushered me into his office – strewn wildly with autopsy slides, microscopes, and tractor drawings by his two young children. He immediately told me of his family, his cattle farm, and his involvement in his church. Charles was what the Irish call a *seannachie*, a storyteller. I thought, 'Who better to deal with a grieving family than this kind, gentle, and generous man, who would listen and try to bring peace to a deeply troubled relative?'

This was the beginning of our friendship. One day in 1994, while the two of us were walking to the Office of the Chief Coroner of Ontario for a meeting on SIDS, I reminded Charles of my search for influenza victims and told him that I had found the burial place of seven Spanish flu victims in Svalbard, Norway. I explained that I hoped that he would agree to serve as the pathologist for my planned project. I wanted him because I admired his ethics and his caring. If I was going to ask to disturb someone's final resting place in another country, I wanted the person doing the work to do so with sensitivity. Charles beamed and proudly announced, 'Consider me on board.' The storyteller explained that he was of Norwegian descent; his grandfather, Tobias Nelson, had journeyed from Norway and had actually founded a Norwegian town, Mandel, in Charles's native Saskatchewan. The *seannachie* looked into the distance, 'Norwegian culture gave me so much. This will give me an opportunity to give something back to Norway.'

A few days later I met with Dr Peter Lewin, a staff paediatrician at Sick Kid's, an assistant professor of paediatrics at the University of Toronto and a palaeopathologist. Peter exuded enthusiasm, good humour, and kindness and was just the type of man any mother would want to look after the well-being of her child. It was perhaps because of his good nature that he had previously served as physician to the queen mother and had earned the trust of Native peoples to whom he brought well-deserved acclaim for their beautiful woodland art.

Not only a true gentleman, but also a respected scientist, Peter has been actively involved in medical archaeology since 1966. He pioneered the use of electron microscopy and the latest imaging techniques in this field, including the CT scan. A CT (computed tomography) scan is an x-ray exam that produces special images of the body. These images define the shape, size, and position of internal body parts, allowing for a diagnosis. As a founding member of the International Paleopathology Association, he had recently been involved in a

CT scanning of mummy Djedmaatesankh, a 30–35-year-old Theban woman from the 22nd Dynastry (ninth century BC). Without destroying Djed's priceless funerary case and her elegantly adorned body, the CT scan revealed what lay inside the woman's beautiful casket of red, gold, and orange: linen wrappings, skin, bones, and, finally, her internal organs, which had been removed, embalmed, and then placed back inside her body in small packages. The scan also revealed that 24 of 28 teeth present in her mouth had been exposed right down to the roots. Her widespread dental infection, including an abscess with pus draining through five different sinuses, would have caused her considerable pain and personal distress and possibly killed her.[1]

In 1994 I asked Peter to join my project because he understands that mummies and other buried human bodies are the remains of real people, not mere artifacts for scientific study. My understanding is that throughout the Earth and throughout time, professionals, family, and friends have carefully prepared the deceased; even the Neanderthal, *Homo sapiens neanderthalensis*, of 130,000–35,000 years ago practised deliberate burial.[2] Families expected that the bodies of their relatives would remain entombed forever and would not be unearthed and subsequently viewed by the world. Peter also understands that buried remains are a precious and unique source of information that can help us to understand ourselves, and he believes that we must treat remains with care and respect. Peter graciously accepted my invitation to join the project.

Although I had become well acquainted with Charles Smith and Peter Lewin, I had yet to have the pleasure of meeting Alan Heginbottom of Ottawa, an emeritus scientist with the Geological Survey of Canada and a fellow of the Royal Geographical Society and the Royal Canadian Geographical Society. Although we had never met, Alan and I had been communicating by telephone and fax for months about permafrost. Alan spoke with passion regarding Longyearbyen's layers of permafrost, bore-hole temperatures, and ground-temperature chronologies.

Alan had been active on behalf of Canada in the International Permafrost Association since its founding in 1983. As a result, I knew of his excellent work – over 120 publications and a recent Circum-Arctic Map of Permafrost and Ground Ice Conditions – and I appreciated his enthusiasm. Alan had, in response to my inquiries, worked extensively in ascertaining the ground temperatures in Longyearbyen over the past eighty years for no reward, for no remuneration. I wanted him to be a member of my research team. Alan readily consented to join the team, analyse the permafrost conditions, and supervise the planned excavation.

Other team members were to include Dr Nancy Arden, Dr Nancy Cox, and Dr Brain Mahy, all from the world-famous Centers for Disease Control (CDC) and Prevention in Atlanta, Georgia, who were to maintain a safe working environment during the exhumations of the miners and were to test any samples retrieved from the bodies for fragments of the 1918 Spanish flu virus.

I knew none of CDC's scientists, and they did not know me. However, Dr Mahy was willing to support my project. On 18 October 1995, he communicated, 'I would like to offer our strong support for your investigation in Spitsbergen, Norway. Influenza viruses have been responsible for some of the worst episodes of pandemic disease in recorded history. The possibility remains high that serious pandemic diseases will occur in the future, and more information on the devastating pandemic of 1918 would be invaluable to CDC, the World Health Organization (WHO) and other public health agencies. We fully endorse Dr Duncan in her efforts to find the remains of permafrost victims. We will also be available to test samples in our Influenza Branch as required for this exciting field project.'

Exhuming the miners could be similar to opening Pandora's box. Lifting the coffin lids might unleash a perfectly preserved virus, the 'Satan bug,' on an unsuspecting, unprepared planet. Every safety precaution would have to be taken, and safety planning would require demanding laboratory and engineering expertise. Who better to provide such safety knowledge than the CDC, with its staff of over 1,000 people identifying, investigating, diagnosing, preventing, and controlling worldwide a wide variety of infectious diseases, such as AIDS, rabies, and ebola? CDC was one of only two labs in North America, and one of only a handful in the world, to house a Biosafety Level 4 (BSL 4) – the ultimate facility for protecting staff and environment from deadly pathogens with which employees work, and for which there are no effective vaccines.[3]

CDC's BSL 4 laboratory has an elaborate air-flow system, increasingly negative pressure in inner rooms, and sealed walls, floors, and ceilings. Its doors have pneumatic rubber seals to render them airtight, and exit air is HEPA-filtered twice. To enter the high security lab, a staff member must don laboratory clothing and a full-body pressurized 'space suit,' which is connected by a hose to an air system. Within the laboratory, people work with infectious organisms using the same kinds of biocontainment equipment and safety procedures as are used in other laboratories, such as BSL 3s. However, the space suit enhances the high level of containment regularly practised.[3]

The final members of the research team were scientists interested in encephalitis lethargica and its possible link with Spanish flu. It was an impressive group comprising: Dr Susan Daniel of the United Kingdom's Parkinson's Disease Society Brain Bank in London; Dr Patrick McGeer, University of British Columbia, Vancouver, Canada; and Dr Daniel Perl and Dr Melvin Yahr, Mount Sinai Hospital, New York.

In August 1994, Dr Perl wrote me, 'I consider the idea of identifying and exhuming affected individuals buried in the permafrost an excellent one, although I am still not entirely convinced that the particular RNAs being sought would remain sufficiently intact over these many years. Nevertheless, I think this is worth pursuing and I would definitely be interested in participating in the research.' In the same month, Dr Yahr informed me, 'The project you propose is of particular interest to me, and I should be delighted to participate as a member of the research team ... The material you propose to obtain is most unique." Finally, as Dr Oliver Sacks, author of *Awakenings*, wrote to me in 1995, my planned project would perhaps 'provide answers to questions we had all given up any hope of seeing answered' – answers to Spanish flu and answers to encephalitis lethargica.

I had assembled a team of experts, leaders in their respective fields, from geology to virology, from three countries, Canada, England, and the United States. The project had clearly required a multidisciplinary research team. I had wanted a multinational team, since flu had raged in Europe, North America, Asia, and elsewhere. I had wanted the team to reflect the global nature of the disease.

Request for Permission, November 1995

With a first-class group of scientists lined up to work with me, on 4 November 1995 I requested permission to undertake my research from the governor of Svalbard, making the promise that Norwegian scientists would be involved throughout the planning and undertaking of the work. I was hoping to invite the Norse Polar Institute to join the project, as the institute had been a key resource in locating the diaries and in answering numerous questions about burial practices in Svalbard and about the depth and extent of permafrost throughout the archipelago.

November passed. And then December sped by, while the Norwegian authorities, as I learned later, debated the merits and drawbacks of the work and questioned whether the project should take place at all. I understood their dilemma. I had asked numerous questions of myself and of my family on finding the location of the young men's graves. Who should speak for the miners? Were there living family members? Should relatives be asked to consent? The young men had, after all, been laid to rest by the community of Longyearbyen and had not been transported back to their native Norway. Is it ethically right to disturb a cemetery? How would the local church rule on the moral dilemma – to exhume the deceased, potentially to help others? How would the nearby community feel about its protected, historical, sacred site being disturbed? Could the work be done safely? Were there any guarantees that nothing deadly would be unleashed?

In late December, I offered to go to Longyearbyen in order to assure the governor, the local church, and the community that the project would involve the highest safety standards and respect and dignity for the deceased. It was crucial that the people of Svalbard and of Norway know that this project was not merely a scientific quest. Rather, it was about seven young men who had died tragically, like tens of millions of others in the world's worst pandemic. It was also important that I become a part of the local community, not just an absentee researcher. The governor's aide, Mr Rolfe Gaarde, however, did not think such a trip necessary at the time. He said, 'Perhaps you could come if we come closer to a decision.'

Norwegian Addition

While the authorities considered whether the project should go forward or not, I received a long fax from a Professor Lars Haaheim, University of Bergen, on Saturday, 25 January 1996. He began, 'I should introduce myself to you, since my name has probably surfaced a couple of times recently ... I think the idea of recovering traces of Spanish Influenza is one I for some time have had myself (although I never got the idea of going to Svalbard. Strangely enough, I went to Longyearbyen last midsummer for a 3–day weekend holiday with my wife. I photographed the gravesite in question without thinking of reading

carefully the dates on the posts!)' Haaheim continued, 'I was first introduced to the outline of your project last fall during my conversations
with Nancy Cox (and later also with Dr Brian Mahy at the CDC) ... I
have communicated with them on several occasions ... So far, I have
not seen the proposal and any background material that has been sent
to the Governor.' He advised me: 'as pointed out in the letter from
Prof. Terje Traavik in Tromso, a Norwegian virologist/microbiologist
should be included as well. Since my name, as Director of the WHO
Influenza Centre of Western Norway, was put forward by Prof. Traavik, I feel that this is a point to consider for you.' Delicacy was essential: 'I should put this as kindly as I can. When approaching "locals,"
be it in Africa or in Norway, a good working relationship with national
expertise is essential. There may be cultural differences that "foreign-
ers" do not appreciate. Like the project of exhuming bodies that have
rested in peace for more than 70 years in a graveyard that can be seen
from large parts of the town. There is no way to "hide" these activities,
of course, no vegetation to help discretion. A good working relationship with townspeople is an absolute must. Also, noisy machinery in a
graveyard which is in use today.' Rolfe Gaarde, the governor's aide,
suggested that Haaheim go to Svalbard to present 'a seminar on influenza in general, the Spanish influenza in particular. And to give some
reassurance about the "seriousness" of the project and the institutions
involved.' Haaheim concluded: 'The angle of Parkinsonism is not a
good one. More importantly, the safety aspects should not be covered
up. The press will smell a rat when they see one. Bringing out a safe
deposit, literally, a virus of apocalyptic potential, is not something one
should handle lightly.'

Haaheim also sent me a copy of his earlier letter to CDC. 'I have
mentioned to you earlier that we have here in Bergen tried to get hold
of specimens from our Pathology Department dating back to the 1918–
20 era. It looked initially very promising, their written records mentioned registration numbers for a range of specimens from diseased
patients from that time. Unfortunately, when they should be recovered
physically, they were gone. Probably missed, or rather thrown away,
during the moves when the new hospital was built in the 70'ties. I was
very surprised that there might be possibilities on Svalbard. And
indeed, I would certainly like to join the project. If you don't mind I
would very much like to get in contact with Dr Duncan.'

I called Haaheim in Bergen immediately and explained that his
name had never surfaced. For three years, I had worked alone and pri-

vately. CDC had recently become involved (and in name only) and was discussing the project openly. Moreover, CDC had invited Haaheim to join my project. And the latter, who had not seen my permission request to the governor, was suggesting appointment of Norwegian scientists, the importance of safety, and the exclusion of encephalitis lethargica.

I explained to Haaheim that I did not appreciate decisions being taken without my consultation. He said, 'Rest safely, no one will take it away from you. There is no chance of your losing control.' He informed me that the governor of Svalbard had appointed him to my research team. He then invited me to go to Longyearbyen with him on 8 February 1996, to discuss my project, of which he knew almost nothing, with the people of Longyearbyen.

I immediately phoned my department head at the University of Windsor, Professor Alan Trenhaile, and explained what had taken place. He volunteered to arrange meetings with our dean, vice-president, and university lawyer so that I could stake a claim on my work and get funding for travel to Longyearbyen.

On 28 January 1996, I faxed CDC to establish a suitable reporting structure. 'I understand that you both ... discussed my project last fall with Professor Lars Haaheim and have been in contact with him more recently. I very much appreciate that you both have excellent contacts and that we should use them. I would, however, have thought that you would have discussed these contacts with me, as I am the project leader. I would require that all contacts be discussed with me. I would also require that my project not be discussed outside the research group. I have been extremely up front with my work: that is, finding seven bodies in permafrost and putting together a first-class research team over the past 2 years. I would very much have liked to have heard of Professor Haaheim.' Brian Mahy called and apologized.

Longyearbyen, April–May 1996

The trip to Longyearbyen that Lars Haaheim suggested that he and I take was repeatedly delayed and eventually abandoned. However, on 26 April 1996, Rolfe Gaarde, on behalf of the governor, invited me to Longyearbyen after surviving family members of the seven miners consented to my project. I was overwhelmed. The families had said 'yes' to a very difficult question and to a stranger half-way around the world. I wondered how many people would have agreed to such a request.

Gaarde invited me to stay at his official government residence. I would be provided with both food and lodging. I politely turned him down, as I did not want to impose, and he had been so kind in answering my numerous questions over the previous six months. He, however, insisted. And eventually, remembering Haaheim's words about approaching locals, I relented, reluctant to offend the governor or her aide.

I was going to the Arctic! At last, I would meet in Longyearbyen the people with whom I had been communicating for so long – Mork, the school teacher, the folks at the Norse Polar Institute, and Gaarde, the governor's aide.

I had less than a week to prepare my plea to the people of Svalbard, to pack, and to arrange for letters and greetings from the two universities for which I work – Windsor and Toronto, where I am an adjunct professor of medical geography. I obtained letters from municipal, provincial, and federal politicians as well.

And then I was on my way to Oslo, Norway, with a brief stop-over in London. From Britain's capital, I took a short flight over Norway's magnificent fjords and snow-laden conifers to Oslo at 59°55" N – as far north as Anchorage, Alaska.[4] A three-hour plane trip carried me north, with a brief stop-over in Tromso, to Longyearbyen, latitude 78° N. At last, the final resting place of the miners. Rolfe Gaarde greeted me and guided me into his car. I was looking forward to the drive, since the flight had proven spectacular over snow-capped mountains, glistening glaciers, and trekking whales in Arctic seas.

We drove the ring road of Longyearbyen. Gaarde remarked on the places of interest. 'UNIS' (University Courses on Svalbard). 'The school, where your Mr Mork works. The glacier. Your cemetery. The church. The church is worried about your project.' He explained that the government residence was not available and that I would be responsible for my own accommodation and food – and so, suddenly, I had new expenses. He, however, would find a place for me to stay. We had dinner in a large cafeteria where the miners were dining, and then Gaarde drove me to my lodging, a room in a long, low, multi-room building.

The next morning I rose early. And with a community map and gifts from Canada in hand, I set off to meet Longyearbyen! My first order of business was to meet Mr Mork, the school teacher, a true bearded Viking at well over six feet tall. Mork welcomed me and introduced me to his principal, Mr Holm, and the other staff members. I thanked him for all the work that he had done on my behalf and presented him with gifts from Canada and with Canadian pins and flags for his students. It was a short visit, as recess was ending. We promised to meet again later. Mork warned me about keeping a lookout for polar bears. Apparently, a person had once been killed immediately outside the restaurant in which Gaarde and I had dined the night before.

Next, I was off to the Norse Polar Institute, SNSK (the coal company), the Svalbard Museum, and UNIS to meet with the instructors regarding their possible involvement in my planned work. I wanted to meet with community leaders and major businesses in order to gain the trust of the people and assure them that our work would be done correctly.

In the afternoon, I met Governor Ann-Kristin Olsen, an elegant stateswoman. After presenting my gifts, I talked at length with her about the project. I was pleased to inform her that Lars Haaheim had joined the project, as her office had requested. The governor was clearly taken aback by my comment: 'Kirsty, we would never tell you whom to have on your team. You have whom you want.' Governor Olsen asked me to stop by the office of *Svalbardposten*, the local newspaper, which claims to be the northernmost paper in the world. She explained that, according to Norway's Freedom of Information Act, all correspondence to and from public offices is open for all to see, including the press. *Svalbardposten* had known of my arrival and wanted to meet with me. And I would have a chance to meet more people from the community through Olsen's invitation to dinner that night at her residence.

After a brief interview with *Svalbardposten*, I walked across the valley floor, which had grazing caribou, to Svalbard Kirke. This was the visit that I had been dreading. I was so afraid that my project would offend the congregation. I knocked at the door of Pastor Jan Hoifodt, the new minister; I had previously been corresponding with Per Arne Engdal. Hoifodt opened the great wooden door, and I introduced myself, 'My name is Kirsty Duncan.' I then blurted out, 'I hope in no way has my project offended you or the church.'

'No,' he hugged me. 'This is exciting work, and it has to be done.' I was very relieved. I had worried for over a year about the church's response. And Jan Hoifodt was supportive. We spoke of his connection to my home, Toronto, where one of his relatives had been stationed during the Second World War in a section of the city known as 'Little

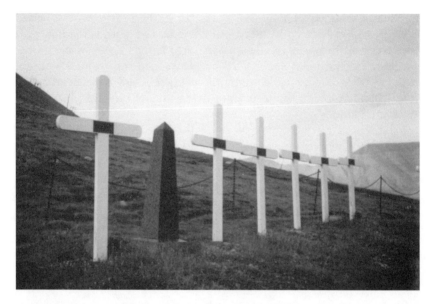

Figure 3   The graves of the seven flu victims.

Norway.' I then gave my host a book on Toronto showing today's Norway Park in the heart of the city.

Jan asked if I was of Norwegian ancestry. He said, 'You know you have a Norwegian name, don't you?'

'I do?'

'Yes, we say, Shoosty.' I liked it; 'Shoosty' sounded friendly (but the Celtic name is pronounced differently in Scotland).

'Have you been to the cemetery?' he asked casually.

'No, I did not think that I had the right to go without your consent.'

'You go. And when you get back, I will take you up on the glacier.'

Sunlight reflected from the snow-covered valley and from the sparkling glacier. And then, high above the valley floor, I saw the white crosses of the cemetery. I climbed slowly up the hill, while reading the names and dates of those buried, until I reached the last and highest row of the little graveyard where the seven miners were buried (Figure 3). I stood motionless in front of their graves. I was the same age – twenty-eight – as the oldest miner when he died.

Did the young men ever imagine that they would lie forever entombed on this barren, windswept slope overlooking the frozen fjord and the white-capped mountains? At their graves, I made a promise to the young miners: to do our work safely and ethically.

After visiting the graves, I returned to Pastor Hoifodt's residence, where my host provided me with the latest in Arctic fashion – a one-piece snowmobile suit with numerous zippers and flaps for protection against the polar wind, snowmobile gloves that extended up to my elbows, and giant snowmobile boots that reached above my knees – for the promised trip to the glacier.

After flying through the town and climbing the cliffs overlooking the cemetery on a giant snow scooter (or snowmobile) with Hoifodt, I met at the governor's soirée many of the people with whom I had spoken earlier in the day, such as Mork, a number of university professors, and the director of SNSK.

About midnight, and under bright skies, I walked back to my lodging, wondering whether I would ever return to Longyearbyen to undertake my project and meet my Arctic friends again. Later that night (in full daylight), I returned to the cemetery around three a.m. to bury a single, long-stemmed yellow rose in the snow under each of the crosses of the seven miners as a symbol of my promise made earlier that day.

Hours later, I left Longyearbyen for Oslo, where at last Lyder Marstrander of the Riksantikvaren (Norwegian Directorate of Cultural Heritage) gave me verbal permission for my project. The trip had been a terrific success. I had permission!

Back in Toronto, on 11 May, I sent a 'Heartfelt Thank You to the People of Longyearbyen' via *Svalbardposten*. I wrote, 'I went to Svalbard in order to first assure you, the people of Longyearbyen, that my project, if allowed, would be undertaken with the greatest respect for the deceased, the families of the deceased, the Office of the Governor, the Church and the people of Longyearbyen. Second, I wanted a greater understanding of the citizens of Longyearbyen and Svalbard itself. Third, I hoped to develop a good working relationship with the Office of the Governor and the people of Longyearbyen. I left Svalbard feeling that you, the people of Longyearbyen, had reassured me. Your kindness, enthusiasm, and encouragement for the project were overwhelming. I left Svalbard with great affection for you, and Svalbard itself; I can hardly wait to return to your enchanting and beautiful Svalbard. Finally, I left Svalbard feeling that I had made new friends. I cannot describe my great feeling of loss when I returned to Oslo. The feeling of loss prevailed because I had left good friends behind in Svalbard.'

4   First Permission, First Workshop

May–August 1996

First Permission, May 1996

Shortly after my return from Longyearbyen, on 15 May 1996, I faxed my team members the news that I had received verbal permission to perform the exhumations. On 16 May, Dr Susan Daniel, the British member, faxed me from London: 'John Oxford has just returned from a meeting in Australia where your project was a major topic. Were you aware of this?' 'Who is John Oxford?' I wondered, and I immediately called Susan to find out. She explained that Professor John Oxford was an influenza virologist working with a friend of hers. Oxford was discussing a 'fantastical project' to recover fragments of the Spanish flu virus from miners' bodies in Spitsbergen and was crediting someone other than me with the idea. Susan, on hearing the news, apparently said, 'Wait, that's Kirsty's project. She started it.' Susan strongly suggested that I do something to get credit for my work.

I immediately called the University of Windsor and told it of my conversation with my British colleague. The university decided to go to the press in order to stake its claim on the work. I felt it necessary to go to the media – but for a very different reason. While I had been planning my project, a big news story burst upon my home city – it was to receive a BSL 4 lab. In fact, the facility had been built with little community involvement.

Why hadn't the community been consulted? What would happen if there was an accident? It appeared to many citizens as if science was above the law, that scientists did not have to proceed through the same permission processes as the general public.

I did not want my project, with its potential risks, being planned in secret. It was important to recognize the risks and weigh the potential benefits. I strongly believed that both the scientific community and the public had the right to debate the project. As a citizen, I would want to know about such a project and would want it carefully monitored.

The ensuing media blitz about the Spitsbergen project was weary-ing. Those who had been through such attention before reassured me that the story would die in a week. It didn't. The interest went on for weeks and weeks; members of the media explained, 'The story has everything doesn't it; the far north, the search for the Satan Bug, and the possibility that something deadly might be unleashed.' There was little peace. In reality, the blitz continued for the next three years, dur-ing which time I received calls from the media almost weekly.

If there had been a great hue and cry against the project, I would have abandoned it. I was, however, inundated by phone calls and per-sonal notes begging for answers about the mysterious Spanish flu. Some elderly people, who had themselves suffered from the disease, called to offer their bodies for research. Their letters and phone calls in particular inspired me to continue working to identify the virus.

While the family phone was ringing off the hook for interviews, I planned to gather the team at the University of Windsor. Following numerous phone calls and faxes, I finally set the Windsor Workshop for 23–24 August 1996, based on the availability of everyone involved, including Professor Lars Haaheim. CDC had provided his available times but had the wrong information. And on May 26th, 1996, Lars requested: 'Since I am one of the influenza experts in the team, in addi-tion to being Norwegian, and having had many conversations with the authorities on this to assist them in their questions, I should very much have liked to be present. I will ask you to contact your partners and see whether a meeting one week later can be arranged.' Since Lars had not in fact been appointed to my team, I was in no hurry to change the dates after everyone else had agreed to them. As a result, the dates of 23–24 August were approved.

Newcomers

When news of my project became known, virologists began calling me, asking to be part of the team. Shortly after Lars's request of late May, one of the world's leading virologists approached me. 'Hello. I am Dr Robert Webster. Young lady, you know who I am, don't you?' He had, he reported, 'been defending my project to everyone all day.' Before I could ask, 'Who is everyone?' and 'Why are you defending my project?' Webster asked to join the team. I had a split second to make up my mind; however, there was no problem deciding, since Webster, professor and chairman of the Department of Virology and Molecular Biology at St Jude Children's Research Hospital, in Memphis, Tennessee, had an international reputation. 'Welcome,' I said.

Webster wrote me on 7 June 1996: 'I greatly appreciate the opportunity to join your research group, for I have spent my entire life working on different aspects of the emergence of pandemic influenza viruses ... Four years ago we spent considerable time in my laboratory ... to analyze the lungs of American soldiers who died in 1918 and whose tissues were stored in formaldehyde since that time.'

A month later, I heard from another virologist, Dr Graeme Laver: 'I expect that you have all the people you need to help you dig, but if you haven't, I would love to help!'

In the weeks leading up to the Windsor meeting in August, most of my correspondence was with documentary makers who wanted the rights to film the expedition. In total, over 300 would ask for the rights. I knew nothing about documentaries, and I knew nothing about regulations and ownership. On 9 July, I received a communication from my university explaining that it wished to help me with a documentary. Dr Julian Cattaneo, vice-president, was 'afraid if you (Kirsty) do not pick a company now, you'll lose the opportunity, and the University will also lose the opportunity.' Cattaneo, after consulting with me, spoke the same day with Elliot Halpern of Associated Producers. It was believed to be a good company; it had, after all, worked with CDC regarding two films on the Ebola virus. On 10 July, Elliot received the rights to cover the project.

On the same day, CDC's Nancy Cox called me. She wanted a bigger team; she wanted to appoint team members, saying that we were lacking expertise in pathology. I, however, set the record straight by explaining that we already had an excellent pathologist – Dr Charles Smith. Nancy then asked that I call those involved in the first or second (1951) expedition to Alaska, such as Dr Jordan and Dr Woodward, for expert advice regarding permafrost exhumations. I contacted the two men, hoping for guidance. Jordan responded with the following words of wisdom, 'They're all dead. No one can help you.' And Woodward said, 'Cox should learn to do her math. I'm old, but not that old' – meaning that he wasn't old enough to have partaken in the Alaskan expeditions of the 1950s.

On 19 July, Brian Mahy and Nancy Cox called me. Both were concerned that Lars Haaheim would not be at the meeting, and could I reschedule it? 'Could the meeting be cut down to just one day? And have you called Dr Woodward?' They then demanded that their pathologist be involved in the project and that no documentary company be present to film the meeting.

I explained patiently that they themselves had given me Haaheim's availability dates, which were incorrect. The conference was about one month away, and I could not in good faith ask team members to cancel flights and accommodation bookings and lose their money; and I further explained that CDC had previously thought that a two-day agenda was reasonable. I relayed Woodward's response, and I repeated that the team already had a top-notch pathologist in Charles Smith. And I agreed to their request that a documentary company not film the conference.

On 8 August, Brian Mahy faxed me. 'We understand your concerns, and if the meeting is still going ahead we need to be there. Nancy Cox, Sherif Zaki and I will arrive ... He is a pathologist who could be invaluable to this project.' I immediately faxed Brian back to say once again that we already had an invaluable pathologist and that Zaki was not needed.

I expected problems at the Windsor meeting. CDC did not like the agenda. CDC wanted another pathologist. And CDC was disappointed that Lars Haaheim was not coming. Also, most of the scientists had never met each other before. My relatively young age would likely be an issue for some members – as it was with the media.

I relayed the expected problems to my university, which suggested a grand opening ceremony, including the Norwegian ambassador, city and provincial dignitaries, and the president of the university, to show that the 'University of Windsor can lead a world-class project.'

My last task prior to the meeting was to learn more about the previous expeditions to Alaska. I spoke with Professor Arnold Monto of the University of Michigan regarding the U.S. army's classified Project George, undertaken by Walter Reed Army Medical Center, Harvard University, and the University of Michigan, with co-operation from the 'Alaskan Brotherhood, the Eskimos.' According to Monto, the research team included 'Ellington, Simmons (dead), Davenport, Hilleman, Murray (dead), Jack Snyder, and 18 troops for protection. A total of 15 bodies from Nome, Soloman, Gulliver, and other Alaskan sites were exhumed, and samples were taken from their lungs for analysis.'

Monto thought it 'definitely worth undertaking the exhumations in Spitsbergen.' 'Even if the body is frozen, it is still a biohazard. Use a negative pressure tent, gloves, dry ice, and put the samples directly in a freezer.' I asked if the army had used any protective safety measures. He responded, 'No protective measures were taken. They didn't even quarantine the area. The Eskimos even looked in the graves. The bodies were grey like charcoal and their cavities empty.' He told me that there was a second expedition and that 'the meat was pink as opposed to Hilleman's grey meat.' He didn't think that either expedition was ever recorded.

Despite this, on 19 August, I spoke and wrote to the U.S. armed forces' archivist, Richard Boylan, regarding the history of the Armed Forces Commission on Influenza, and specifically Project George. He found no reference to the project.

Shortly thereafter, I secured from Dr Peter Jahrling, a biosafety expert from the U.S. Army Medical Research Institute of Infectious Diseases (USAMRIID), a copy of an e-mail sent by A.S. Beneson. It discussed a very different Project George. 'In 1984, I wrote to Jack (John C.) Snyder at Harvard after hearing a rumour that he and Ed Murray had isolated influenza virus from bodies in the permafrost. His answer, dated Jan 31, 1984 was: "Ed Murray, Fred Davenport, Maurie Hilleman and several others flew in an Air Force DC3 to Nome, Alaska, circa Sept. 1950 under General Simmons. We set up an elaborate isolation station to handle specimens. Dry ice, etc, pyrex ampoules for division of tissues to Walter Reed, Harvard, Michigan labs. Mass graves were found – we had permission to exhume from the Eskimo Brotherhood."'

The results were disappointing. 'NO, repeat, NO influenza viruses (or other pathogens except a few staph aureus) were recovered by any of us. We judged from the physical appearance of the bodies and tissues that the permafrost level had moved up and down a few times during the interval from 1918 (when the bodies were buried) and 1950 when exhumed ... It was exciting – we gave the project a really good try – chick embryos, x-rayed cotton rats, mice, even ferrets, and several routes of inoculation for each, to no avail. Al Coons tried fluorescent antibody (but his reagents at that time were, in his own words, much too crude to shed real light on the question).'

I immediately called Walter Reed, Harvard, and Michigan, to ask if samples existed from the classified expedition. The answer was 'No.'

My final calls before the workshop were to Dr Peter Jahrling, USAMRIID. Jahrling answered, 'So, you're the flu lady. Great project.' I replied: 'I'm glad you think so. We need a biosafety expert. CDC is involved, but I want a true biosafety expert. Would you like to be involved? We're having a conference in a few days; perhaps you could attend.' 'I'd love to on all counts.'

On 19 August, I faxed Jahrling a synopsis of the project and information regarding the conference. On the 21st, I received a polite letter from him explaining that it would not be appropriate for his lab to participate and that he could not attend the workshop. 'As a group, we are very interested in this project and would like to see it succeed. We are also happy to offer our scientific expertise and to lend our BSL 4 facilities to the effort if asked. From your perspective, one potential downside of enlisting USAMRIID collaboration would be the perception that isolation of the 1918 influenza strain has sinister (i.e. biological warfare) overtones ... It would not be appropriate for us to participate, however, unless CDC invited us to do so. I spoke with Dr Mahy this morning, and he indicated that if samples were obtained and BSL 4 containment facilities were required, that CDC would be able to meet that demand.' That is, CDC would work alone – without USAMRIID's help – unless CDC specifically asked for assistance.

I immediately called Jahrling, who had been so keen to participate, and asked why the change of heart. 'CDC has shut me down.' He repeated, 'CDC has shut me down.' How could another institution prevent his involvement in a meeting? He did not elaborate. However, he said that he would like to be kept informed of developments and that he would keep me abreast of any relevant information from his end. I promised to send him the conference proceedings.

Windsor Workshop, August 1996

23 August 1996. At last, I would meet my team. Relations had thus far been difficult. I knew that the university, eager for publicity, would have the press out in full force. I needed quiet time to think of the science. I did not need any distractions, such as Elliot Halpern and his film crew. I had promised CDC that there would be no filming. Elliot had been pushing relentlessly but I refused. I had promised no filming and no contract had been signed. Elliot then asked permission of my university without informing me. A former lawyer, he understood that I was merely an employee and that the university would want the press coverage. The university consented.

I told Elliot that he could film only the opening ceremony, not the scientific meeting. Thus I would keep my word to CDC. However, unbeknown to me, Elliot had also called CDC and sought permission to film from CDC's public relations people, who also consented. Associated Producers (AP) was permitted to film, and all team members except me signed the mandatory release form, permitting the company to use the film footage and images. When AP arrived in Longyearbyen in August 1998 to film phase II – the exhumations – I did sign its release because Norway required that I grant open access to the media; however, I wrote a clear proviso on the form that the company could not use my image in the Windsor film footage. After viewing the documentary, aired in February 1999, I immediately called my lawyer: 'I wrote a proviso. How can he get away with it (using the Windsor film footage)?' 'Kirsty, Elliot was a lawyer, and he knows how to get around the rules. Elliot knows that you could try to prevent the show from being aired. But if you do, there will be a hue and cry against you and your project. Elliot will claim that you are trying to stop public knowledge, and in the end, more people will watch the documentary because of the publicity you generated.' 'What would you do?' 'My advice: nothing.'

The first order of business of the scientific meeting was mine: to introduce all the team members to each other and to describe what expertise each person brought to the table. The planned project was multidisciplinary and needed the geographer's initial detective work, the geologist's interpretation of permafrost conditions, and the pathologist's retrieving of samples. Virology was the final phase of the project. If the exhumations did not yield samples, there would be no virology. Unfortunately, they were unable to understand or respect the expertise of the other disciplines. Repeatedly, the virologists maintained, 'A geologist could never understand what a virologist does.'

Regardless, geologist Alan Heginbottom discussed permafrost conditions at Longyearbyen, digging conditions, and digging requirements. Alan, an excellent teacher, had even brought his home-made permafrost so that laboratory scientists could understand field conditions. Robert Webster stated that he was greatly concerned because the presence of permafrost might mean that the virus was viable. Webster said that we would have to be conscious of the risk from the very beginning and that we would have to investigate methods of looking at the body and containment of the virus so that contamination of the environment would not occur. Robert was adamant that we did not want a live virus and we should just go for the genetic material.[1]

I asked Brian Mahy to comment on potential danger. He said that

there might be a chance, perhaps 5 per cent, that the virus would be viable. Therefore every precaution would have to be taken: for example,
negative pressure tents. If the samples were kept frozen, the danger
would lie in removing them. I then asked Mahy if he was confident that
the project could be undertaken safely. 'Yes,' he said emphatically. 'We
just have to take adequate precautions.'[1]

Next, Charles Smith and Peter Lewin explained their ideas. Charles
said that the first and cardinal rule of exhumation is simply: 'You don't
know what you will find until you look." Smith explained that many
variables can affect a body's preservation and that it is simply not possible to predict the state of preservation prior to performing an exhumation. Sometimes, he said, unpleasant surprises occur in exhumation, and sometimes there is unexpectedly good preservation. He then
spoke of the two classical autopsy techniques: the Virchow or modified
Virchow, which requires that 'the organs be removed from the body
either one at a time or in groups'; and the von Rokitansky, which
requires that the entire thoracic and abdominal contents be removed
en bloc and dissected. Dr Smith explained that neither minimizes
infection.[1]

Instead, both Smith and Lewin suggested using a hollow coring
device, similar to those used to sample trees, to remove a long, slender
core of flesh. The device could be fashioned so as to produce neither
heat nor aerosol that might allow the spread of infection. Finally, Smith
discussed personnel for the autopsy, and techniques for restoring both
the coffins and the cemetery after the exhumations.[1]

Next, CDC's Nancy Cox talked at length about the influenza pandemic of 1918. Dr Daniel Perl, a neuropathologist, suggested that if the
team wanted archival tissue samples, he could provide contacts with
the Mayo Clinic, which keeps all tissue samples.'[1]

Brian Mahy explained what scientific resources CDC was willing to
make available. He said that 'CDC makes a unique offering – the finest
maximum-containment lab. There are others, but not as large or easy
to use. CDC can work safely with many infectious agents without fear
of contamination in a level 4 lab.' For the future site, Brian offered
'full/half protection suits in negative pressure tents.'[1]

It was agreed that testing of any samples would be done in a BSL 4
lab and that CDC would require independent confirmation of results
by other labs: the BSL 4 laboratories at USAMRIID, and in Winnipeg,
Manitoba, Canada. Prior to sharing the samples, however, the team
would have to make sure that no live virus was recovered.[1]

Finally, Daniel Perl discussed the possible relation of encephalitis lethargica to the influenza of 1918. He had offered to present evidence or a possible link, but at the meeting he suggested that the two were probably unrelated. He said that it might be purely coincidence that Spanish flu and encephalitis lethargica happened at the same time. The literature was inconclusive.[1]

To close the day's meeting, I asked each team member for comments. Brian Mahy said that he could not imagine how to deal with the possible link with encephalitis lethargica; we might learn more about the 1918 flu by looking at tissue already available from around the world. But he did like 'the glamour of digging up bodies.' He suggested that the team be more aggressive in trying to locate archival tissue – perhaps from the Mayo Clinic. Nancy Arden of CDC thought the idea of exhuming bodies intriguing, but she agreed with Brian: 'Instead of pursuing risky exhumation, the team should consider other ways of answering questions.'[1]

Charles Smith believed that we should go ahead with the project but suggested a two-pronged approach of using archival samples and the proposed frozen samples from Spitsbergen. He thought that encephalitis lethargica could be a later, spin-off project. Rob Webster thought that the team should 'pursue all avenues.' Daniel Perl found the idea of retrieving archival material intriguing. He offered to make initial calls to the Mayo Clinic and Johns Hopkins.[1]

Back at the hotel, I summarized the day's events, noting contradictions between earlier comments and what was said at the meeting. I needed a game plan. Either the team wanted to proceed with Splitsbergen, or it did not. Either way, I needed a decision. If the group wanted to proceed, I needed to draw it together, or, as Dr Smith so eloquently stated, I needed to 'herd the cats.' 'Cats,' added Charles, 'are generally solitary animals, who do not herd easily.'

24 August 1996. I gambled. 'Good morning,' I read from my prepared statement. 'I am shocked and disappointed by some of your final comments. For two years, some of you have expressed great interest and enthusiasm for this field project. Suddenly, we are talking about archival material. The purpose of this workshop was to discuss the nuts and bolts of the field project – how to make the project work. I don't feel that we can go any further until we get some things straight. As your host, I find this very difficult to say – but if you are not committed to the field project, I will have to ask you to leave.'

There was a brief silence. The world's flu experts had not expected such an ultimatum from a geographer – a non-scientist, in the virologists' eyes. I continued, 'I am asking who is committed ... I've worked 3½ years on this.'[2]

Robert Webster responded, 'And I have worked a lifetime, my young lady. You're a neophyte in this area. None of us want to take what you've achieved.'[2]

'I would not want to impose, as a neophyte, my views on you,' I responded quietly.[2]

The disturbance blew over. Everyone agreed to stay. Nancy Cox said, 'There has been some misunderstanding. Scientifically, this project has always been interesting.' She finished by saying that CDC would be responsible for most finances.[1]

'Nancy, thank you ... Perhaps we should break into the two working groups (an exhumation group and a virological group).'[1]

The virologists, along with Daniel Perl, went to their assigned room to discuss laboratory analyses, and the Canadians, all part of the same exhumation working group, relaxed. The plan had worked! The virologists had committed themselves! Charles Smith just kept saying, 'You did it! You did it! No one left.'

At the end of the two meetings, the team reunited. CDC, Daniel Perl, and Rob Webster returned with an outline of how to undertake the exhumation work safely. The virologists finally wanted to talk about Svalbard, and they wanted to proceed with the project as planned.

The team agreed to treat the site as potentially dangerous. The work area would require a negative-pressure tent with shower facilities, and the workers, full protective gear, prophylactic treatment, and influenza vaccines. The virologists would need a minimum of three samples from seven organs in each body. The samples would be analysed at two separate labs, each performing the tests independently and agreeing on the results before releasing them. The budget would include $50,000 per lab for the treatment and handling of samples and $250,000 for transportation of samples. CDC, however, had an agreement with the U.S. air force regarding transportation, and it was thought that 'the costs could be absorbed.' In total, it was thought that about $500,000 would be required.[1]

Since we comprised a multi-agency group, geologist Alan Heginbottom and virologist Robert Webster requested a formal agreement, a memorandum of understanding, by which team members would agree to abide.

Brian Mahy suggested dropping the experts on encephalitis lethargica, as they did not seem to be able to contribute meaningfully at that time. Daniel Perl thought that that was 'okay, as long as we get to sample any brain material.' I strongly disagreed with letting go of committed colleagues. I explained that the encephalitis people were involved first, and no decisions could be made regarding their future involvement.[1]

The meeting at last drew to a close. Robert Webster concluded, 'It is very exciting that the project has progressed this far and that Kirsty Duncan has pending approval' for the exhumations. The team members agreed to continue planning for Spitsbergen so that the project could begin once written permission was granted. And they also agreed to search in the meantime for archival material preserved in formalin. The more samples, the better![1] A new hunt for archival samples began.

5 Archival Samples? CDC Withdraws

August 1996 – June 1997

Three Sets of Samples?

Despite the initial trials of the team's first workshop, everyone seemed to be on side when the meeting at last adjourned. We all agreed on continued planning and an archival search. I wondered, however, what would happen. Would momentum of the first meeting continue? Or would the team members quietly realign themselves or drift away?

On 28 August 1996, Rob Webster faxed support: 'It is apparent from the meeting that this project will be very complex and involve a great deal of protocol preparation and biosecurity. Of uppermost importance is the protection of personnel and the environment against the possibility of contamination ... any possibility at all means that strict biosecurity must be used throughout the project.'

I next received Daniel Perl's communiqué of 6 September: 'At the meeting I volunteered to find archival Spanish flu tissue samples ... Based on a few telephone calls, it seems that I will be able to identify preserved pathology tissue samples from the 1918 epidemic. This obviously does not preclude our efforts.' Webster and Perl, the neuropathologist who wanted encephalitis lethargica dropped, clearly wanted to go forward. In fact, on 6 September, Daniel called me to inform me that he was able to locate at least twenty tissue samples; he did not share the source. The project was gaining speed.

I faxed Daniel on 7 September: 'I look forward to receiving information about these samples in the near future.' On 28 September, I again asked him about the tissue. On 15 November I faxed him for a third time: 'In your letter of September 6th, 1996, and our telephone call of September 6th, 1996, you mentioned your finding preserved pathology samples from the 1918 epidemic. In our September 6th conversation, you said that you were able to locate at least 20 tissue samples. As the team agreed to information sharing, I require information about the samples in order to pass on information to the rest of the team. I did ask for the information regarding the samples in my letters of September 7th, 1996, and September 28th, 1996, to you.' Still no response. On 18 February, I faxed Daniel for a fourth time – again to no avail.

On 21 March 1997, I took a different tack. I phoned Daniel and apparently caught him off guard. He said, 'I didn't know it was you.'

'I know, I didn't give my name.'

He stumbled briefly, before blurting out, 'I've already spoken to Nancy [Cox].'

'About what?

'The samples.'

'Good. Could you tell me what's happening? And will you be able to attend the team's upcoming meeting at CDC?' (finally scheduled for 8 April).' Daniel reluctantly answered my questions. He had indeed found samples (although he would not say from where), and he couldn't attend the team's second workshop at CDC.

I immediately faxed Nancy Cox: 'I just spoke with Daniel Perl. He explained that he contacted you this morning regarding the ~20 influenza tissue samples (mentioned in his September 6th, 1996, letter to me) and an unspecified number of encephalitis lethargica samples. I think that the finds are extremely exciting. I am disappointed that Daniel is unable to make the meeting (at CDC on April 8th). He explained, however, that he will be meeting with you a week later in Atlanta. I was wondering if CDC might be able to provide a telephone hook-up to Daniel in Guam. Daniel said that he would be willing to be available for a hook-up.'

Daniel was planning to meet privately with Nancy the following week. I did not like the idea of a private meeting, which might produce a spin-off project. As a result, I had Daniel agree to a telephone call from Guam so that he could openly discuss the promised samples with the team. I then had Nancy agree to arrange the call to include Daniel in the meeting.

Because the team had agreed to search for tissues preserved in formalin, I too diligently pursued archival samples. On 16 October 1996, I called Dr Peter Jahrling of USAMRIID, the biosafety scientist who had wanted to attend the Windsor Workshop. Jahrling offered to make some phone calls regarding the army's classified expedition to Alaska and any resulting samples.

He also informed me that he might be working with the Russians to find victims of the Spanish flu buried in the Siberian permafrost.

Later the same day, he faxed me: 'Looked over my notes from the Swords into Plowshares meeting. "While there was interest expressed on the U.S. side regarding an expedition to find flu in the permafrost, there was also correspondence from the Russians which pointed out that 1918 was the middle of the Russian revolution; thus burial records and the like were not available ... The issue is not dead; our delegation will suggest that the Russians consider this once again."'

On 15 November, I faxed Peter Jahrling requesting any news. On 22 November, he explained, 'There has not been any specific movement with regard to the Russian initiative to search for flu victims in the permafrost, but I can tell you that there are several U.S. initiatives ... so I expect to see some concrete proposals soon ... I will share whatever information I can with you, and hope that it leads to something substantial.'

I spoke with Nancy Cox in February 1997, regarding the Siberian effort. She reported, 'The records were not kept as well organized as those for the Svalbard bodies. The project is not viewed as a strong project by CDC.'

While communicating with Peter Jahrling, I learned from our team's geologist, Alan Heginbottom, of Professor John Oxford's work, using archival samples to examine the proposed link between Spanish flu and encephalitis lethargica. While visiting family in England, Alan had read an article about Oxford's research in a British newspaper. Oxford had previously heard of my work at the meeting in Australia, where someone else was taking credit for my work.

I first wrote to Oxford on 18 October 1996. After receiving no response, I called him on 8 November, and we discussed our mutual research interests. I followed up with a fax. 'I was delighted to learn of your exciting work. I was especially delighted to hear that you would be interested in participating in my project (using archival and permafrost samples to identify the 1918 influenza) ... How do we convince the flu experts that a possible link between influenza and encephalitis lethargica is important and worthy of study?' John responded to my fax on the same day. 'As regards Von Economo's disease I find this a particularly relevant aspect because circumstantial and epidemiological evidence, some reported from the CDC, support the idea of causation by influenza ... I feel strongly that we need to know whether certain pandemic influenza viruses have a degree of neurotropism ... However they may not be familiar with the early literature on the subject.' John reported 'interest from an eminent neurologist [name not given], now 97 years old, who probably is the last person alive who diagnosed such cases in the 1920's ... There are not many groups working in this area which seems very important to me (John Oxford). Also it is the sort of work that needs an international team of experts with a wide range of disciplines. We both seem to be near accomplishing that and it might help to join forces.'

A week later I began arranging finances to travel to London to meet with Oxford. On 4 December I heard from Lyder Marstrander of Norway's Directorate of Cultural Heritage: 'Lars [Haaheim] is a bit concerned that the Parkinson disease is getting too much attention from the project compared with the Spanish flu.' On 6 December, I tried to calm Lars: 'Regarding the question of encephalitis lethargica: the Spanish flu question must be answered first. Encephalitis lethargica is a second question.'

I met John Oxford, professor of virology, in London on 3 February 1997. He appeared the English academic in a blue sports jacket complete with elbow patches and grey scarf. He and his friend Dr Rod Daniels of the National Institute for Medical Research (NIMR) were expecting someone older. At first, Oxford volunteered nothing, he offered nothing. He even appeared to forget his previous suggestion of our joining forces. In order to make sure that these two men would not ignore me, I flew into work mode, and I excitedly discussed the science. And suddenly, John showed great enthusiasm. He wanted to know everything. He wanted to know the 'players,' and he began to 'guess' some of the troubles. He seemed to know intimately the inner workings of the team. But how was that possible?

I didn't want to discuss politics. But he understood. He said, 'CDC can be difficult. They like to run the show.' These were precisely Jahrling's words during two phone calls. Oxford asked me why I planned to dig in Spitsbergen. He asked why I hadn't looked closer to home. I said, 'I have a back-up site – Labrador. I do not want to have to resort to the Canadian site though, as it is an Aboriginal site. Permission to exhume would be extremely difficult.' His face clouded momentarily. He asked sharply, 'What do you know about Labrador? I know about Labrador.' He continued, 'A Canadian wrote to me and told me about a burial pit in Labrador.' But that's all Oxford knew about Spanish influenza in Canada.

I filled him in on the details of the last days of the 1918 influenza outbreak in Okak, Labrador. He then suggested, 'Perhaps we could work there together. The Labrador missionaries were associated with my university. The link would probably get us permission.' I did not think so.

He then proposed that if he and Rod could join my project, he would in return offer his archival samples to the research team. Thus the team would procure samples from both Daniel Perl and from John Oxford. At the end of the day, he showed me a photograph and asked me if I knew the man in the picture. I did not. John proudly announced that the man was his very good friend Lars Haaheim, with whom he and his family often vacationed. I suddenly understood John's inside information – and he confirmed his source.

On 10 February 1997, I phoned Lars Haaheim, who was on sabbatical leave at CDC, and explained that I had met his friend. I further explained that Oxford promised to let us examine his samples if he and Rod Daniels could join our team. I thought that Lars would be pleased. Instead, he was angry. He demanded, 'Why did you contact John Oxford? He can't contribute anything. We do not need any hangers-on.' I was surprised, since John had spoken so highly of him.

On 20 February, I received a letter from John Oxford. 'I enjoyed ... catching your enthusiasm, expertise and also your frustrations about the project. It is a very exciting opportunity indeed and also I am sure you will not allow a few small bureaucratic problems to impede the science. It is better to get everyone's support now rather than having them agitating afterwards ... Perhaps Lars has had his feathers ruffled a little because he has done some not inconsiderable work behind the scenes to facilitate permission, etc. As you will see he is better in the flesh than on the phone ... As I know you appreciated it is only a question of making sure everyone has been consulted and not excluded, a little like the Sleeping Beauty story where one person was not invited to the party and later caused problems!'

Oxford concluded: 'Finally I have written to Nancy Cox ... and suggested that we should exchange material, that is, we should send her our lungs (from The Royal Hospital, London, England) and we (Rod Daniels and myself) would wish to have access to material from your excavation. I assume you would be agreeable to this? Incidentally my strong advice is that you should form a *formal* "Scientific Advisory group (SAG)" to report to you as "Principal Investigator." I would advise you to have a senior virology person to chair the SAG and also report to you. Such arrangements are very necessary and ensure that ultimately you are in control and I for one have every confidence in your energy, knowledge and ability to do this.'

The letter was helpful. John Oxford was, yet again, understanding of the bureaucratic tribulations and was trying to smooth relations with Lars Haaheim. If I followed his suggestions, the team would have access to Oxford's archival material, but a SAG is a double-edged sword – providing support, but reducing my direction. (As project leader, I maintained sole control, but with SAG, I would hold only one vote of six.)

I thought that CDC would be elated about access to Oxford's material. John had privately told me that Brian Mahy had previously asked for his samples, but that he had refused him. But now, mainly through my work and outreach, CDC would have access to Oxford's European archival samples.

At this point, in late February 1997, my team was assured of two sets of archival data. Was a third set possible? I had one last opportunity with Dr Albert McKee, one of the Iowa participants in the Alaskan expedition of 1951. I once again contacted McKee on 31 March 1997 to discuss whether his team members – Dr Johan Hultin (McKee's student) and Dr Otto Geist – had tissue samples. McKee seemed uncomfortable talking with me. Perhaps he was afraid that I would make trouble for him because of the lack of safety measures in his 1951 expedition. He kept repeating, 'I don't want any trouble, I don't want any trouble. It was different then, you know? There just weren't the safety standards.' I assured him that causing trouble was not my aim. I just wanted his help, his advice.[1]

McKee gave me a brief recounting of the trip – a description different from the one reported by Dr Hultin in the newspapers in 1997. McKee said that his 'was the first expedition and the "Army" expedition was the second expedition.' He told me that he and his team members (Hultin and Geist) went to Teller Mission, where only 8 of 115 'Eskimos' survived the pandemic. The deaths had occurred so quickly, and there were so many bodies, that the mission called in the U.S. army. The troops used a steam generator to thaw the permafrost before burying the bodies in a common grave.[1]

McKee said that the expedition cost $3000, and that his team received all the necessary permissions from the governor, the state's health commissioner, the teacher (legal representative), and the chief of the village. He said that they 'flew to Alaska, and three people did the exhumations in one day. The lungs were then packed in dry ice in vacuum bottles.'[1] An 'Eskimo' then rowed McKee and the precious lungs back to Nome, where he 're-snowed his packs.' He said that no safety precautions were taken because he 'had been vaccinated against influenza so many times, and with cross-immunity, I was fine.' McKee explained that no one but he would have had the samples, and I already knew that he didn't have any.[1]

My team would still have access to material from Perl and Oxford. I could hardly wait for the team's April meeting at CDC to share the exciting news with everyone.

Written Permission, February 1997

I received initial written notice on 11 January 1997 that Norway's Directorate of Cultural Heritage had granted permission (until 31 December 1997) for the project. I was elated. Fifteen months of waiting was over. I had been given a very great opportunity. I immediately telephoned and then faxed my research team.

Rob Webster was ecstatic. He said, 'We should move right away.' Then, he immediately changed his mind. He would have to talk to Lars Haaheim first to see what he thought about the permission. On 19 January Haaheim wrote. 'The first thing you should bring to their attention is the limited time window given for the project. It will of course be impossible to finish the project at the site within the calendar year!' CDC concurred.

The Canadians, however, were ready. They had continued planning for five months, as we had agreed at the Windsor Workshop. Alan Heginbottom had investigated the pros and cons of using ground-penetrating radar (GPR) to locate the graves. He had also produced draft after draft of detailed excavation plans. Our American colleagues, in contrast, had been waiting for written permission. Alan recommended, 'If we have to do it, let's get on and do it. Perhaps we should dump CDC and just do it with the Canadians.'

Understanding that our U.S. colleagues needed more time, I requested on 19 January 1997 an extension of the permission to 31 December 1998. Permission, however, was denied by Lyder Marstrander in February 1997. I once again faxed my team. 'As you know, permission has been granted until 31 December 1997. I hope that you find this exciting and challenging ... We have to move now. The Norwegian authorities have spent the past 15 months working strenuously on our behalf ... If we do not undertake the project now, Norway will rightly question our credibility and ability. In 1996, descriptions of a total of 146 projects from 17 nations were received in Svalbard. We are extremely fortunate to have been given permission for our project. Norway has done their part; we must now do ours.'

Rob Webster remained supportive. On 6 February 1997 he wrote, 'Thank you ... for the good news ... I am extremely interested in cooperating with you in any way ... Is a follow-up meeting planned now that you have this permission?'

A second meeting was indeed needed. In order to show good faith, I asked if Lars Haaheim would be willing to chair the gathering at CDC. Nancy Cox suggested that Peter Jahrling be involved in the project. CDC had 'shut down' Jahrling the previous August, although I had continued to keep him informed. Needless to say, I was pleased that she now wanted Jahrling on board.

I received final written permission from the Norwegian authorities on 5 February: 'The cemetery of Longyearbyen is a protected monument according ... to the Regulations concerning the Cultural Heritage of Svalbard ... it is forbidden to damage, dig up, change or move any protected monument unless permission has been granted. Since the cemetery is both a protected monument and a cemetery for the Church in Longyearbyen, and since there are living relatives of those buried there, we have given this application a closer consideration than usual.' Several people and institutions had evaluated the project: 'The University of Bergen has strongly supported the application ... The Church Council for Svalbard has no objection to the project. The Diocesan Council for Svalbard also has no objection. The Norwegian Research Council has supported the application ... The Governor of Svalbard has also been in contact by telephone with relatives of two of the deceased. They have no objection to the project.' The directorate believed 'that the project is well founded and important to carry out ... Since it involves a burial ground and not just a cultural monument, the Directorate urges that proper respect be shown to the burials during the fieldwork ... Furthermore we urge that special measures should be taken to shield the site during excavation ... The Directorate is pleased ... that Professor Lars Haaheim, Bergen, has agreed to act as co-ordinator for the Norwegian side.'

The directorate gave me 'permission to exhume 7 bodies from the graveyard of Longyearbyen, Svalbard.' It set a number of conditions: 'The work must be carried out with due respect to the deceased and to the environment (churchyard). No bodies shall be removed from the churchyard, only the necessary samples for analysis. A description of the procedures during fieldwork shall be submitted to the State Health Authorities. The work must be carried out during October or late autumn. No wheeled or tracked machines will be allowed. The work shall be carried out under the supervision of the Governor of Svalbard and those taking part in the project must follow any orders that may be given by the Governor during fieldwork.'

After removal of samples, 'the excavated soil shall be replaced and the surface reconstructed, so that there are no visible traces of the graves having been opened. If a situation should arise that is not covered by these conditions, the Regulations for the Cultural Heritage of Svalbard shall be pursued or the matter presented to the Directorate for final decision. The permission is valid until 31 December 1997. If for some reason the project has not been carried through within that date, a new permission must be applied for.'

I was thankful that so many groups had said 'yes.' A phone call came 'out of the blue' from Mr Marstrander of the directorate on 17 February. I wondered why he was calling. Apparently, Lars Haaheim had called Marstrander to tell him that I was displeased regarding the permission. I said, 'That simply is not true.' I really appreciated what had been done on the Norwegian side. I could not have asked that the permission be handled better. 'Why was Lars Haaheim meddling?' I wondered. He was the one who didn't think that there was sufficient time to do the work and had asked that I request an extension.

I then faxed Marstrander a letter. 'I want you to know that I happily and gratefully accepted the end date for the permission granted on January 16th, 1997. However, my American colleagues wanted an extension of the permission. On their behalf, on 19 January 1997, I asked for an extension of the permission ... My Canadian colleagues and myself would very much have liked to undertake the project this year. Unfortunately, my American colleagues require extra time. I am deeply embarrassed when you, your Office and the people of Svalbard have undertaken so much on our behalf. My sincerest apologies. As promised, I will contact you after our April meeting when I know more about timelines.'

Nancy Cox on 18 February suggested 1 or 4 April for the CDC meeting and asked that I fax the team the choice of dates. She questioned who would fund the project, despite volunteering at our first workshop that CDC would cover costs. On 26 February, Brian Mahy faxed me regarding financing. 'I am sure that you must remember that I never agreed to pay the costs of an expedition to Svalbard, although I did agree that CDC would be able to test samples and cover the costs for this.' I responded the same day quoting the first workshop's minutes. 'She (Nancy Cox) would be responsible for most of the finances.' As well, 'Mahy said that they counted on reducing the costs by $250,000.00 through CDC's contacts with the air force.' Mahy said, 'If PCR (an analytical testing method for viral DNA) is undertaken, CDC would require independent confirmation from other labs ... Finally, CDC should be able to cover costs.'

On 27 February, Nancy suggested new dates for the meeting and again asked that I fax the team. On 6 March, she requested a third date, 8 April, and another team faxing. The day after my last faxing, expressing my own frustration, Charles Smith wrote me, 'I certainly don't know how those folks manage to do any real work if they cannot even set a date for a meeting.'

Shortly thereafter, Nancy Cox and I spoke on the telephone. I explained that I had commitments the night before her meeting and would be unable to fly until the morning of the workshop. I therefore asked if she could start the meeting at 10:30 a.m. She said that she would consider my request and that she would call me back before finalizing the agenda. There was no return call.

On 31 March, CDC faxed a formal invitation to the workshop for 8 April. Since I did not receive the invitation and agenda, I learned of the conference details only from one of my Canadian team members. Nancy apologized for the 'faxing error.'

Partial Answer to Spanish Flu

A fax from Peter Jahrling: 'Congratulations on the progress of your Norway project. I very much appreciate being kept in the loop, and I am very interested in seeing this project succeed. Unfortunately, I have prior commitments (regarding April 8th) ... for a conference in Atlanta.' He told me 'that an article is scheduled for publication in the 7 March (1997) Science, by Taubenberger et al., in which they present the sequence of nine fragments of RNA that were successfully analyzed from paraffin-embedded tissues of 1918 vintage influenza victims. I'm not sure if availability of this information will impact the concerns about biohazard or the paleovirology endeavor, but you should at least be aware of its existence.' Taubenberger's work was a surprise to me. He had, it turned out, obtained samples from the Armed Forces Institute of Pathology. The army, however, had informed me that no samples existed. I was taken aback but pleased at least that someone was actually getting answers.

Charles Smith faxed me a week later. 'Did you know that someone has submitted an article to *Science* in which they have found some of the Spanish flu virus in old archival material? Peter Lewin [also at the Hospital for Sick Children] told me about it this morning. The paper isn't published yet – a journalist phoned him to learn the status of our expedition.'

Nancy Cox called me on 17 March. She suggested that we invite Taubenberger to the team's meeting at CDC. I thought it an excellent idea. We on the team needed to learn of his work to decide whether to proceed with our project.

Two days later, I heard from Gina Kolata, medical reporter for the *New York Times*. She wanted to ask me some questions about the 1918 flu. I gave my stock answer, 'I am sorry, but the team agreed last August not to do any more interviews.' She explained that she would be forced to write that I refused to comment if I didn't answer her questions. I said, 'That would be dishonest.' She posed her question anyway: 'How can you rightly go ahead with the Norway project in light of Taubenberger's work?' A 'no comment' would look as though I was hiding information. I was simply honouring my August agreement with my team. I explained that I would get back to her after communicating with my colleagues.

I spoke with both Brian Mahy and Nancy Cox. We agreed on the following statement. 'The team is getting together in Atlanta, Georgia, in order to discuss the new results (i.e., Dr Taubenberger's work). In fact, we have invited Dr Jeffrey Taubenberger to the meeting. And we will be discussing and debating how to proceed from here.' I read the statement to Gina word for word. I then asked that she read the statement back to me. She read it exactly as I had dictated and promised to send me the article.

Since I did not receive a timely copy of her article, I managed to track it down at the airport. There were several errors in it. Dr Julian Cattaneo, vice-president, University of Windsor, wrote a letter of complaint to the *New York Times* on 25 March pointing out the inaccuracies and omissions, including Gina's failure to mention that we had invited Taubenberger to our meeting.

John Oxford faxed me on 20 March. 'Kirsty, I expect you know that the U.S.A. group (Dr Taubenberger et al.) has a partial sequence from a 1918 sample ... I guess the CDC group might argue that this lessens the need for disinterring in Spitsbergen. So I feel it is important to think of the possible advantages of having those samples. For example: [It] might tell us something the formalin-fixed material does not. It [the Spitsbergen project] might not be dangerous at all. In fact, many of the infectious disease people here are not alarmed ... The cadavers might, in the fullness of time, come to the surface unexpectedly in a thaw and it would be better to know under controlled conditions of our chance, if any, dangers there are.'

John was no longer worried about infection. He had found Dr Susan Young, a pathologist for 'Necropolis, The Mass Exhumation Specialists (it is not uncommon for the company to exhume tens of thousands of human remains in any one year),' and her 'opinion is that the risk of the exhumation especially when frozen is zero' (fax of 25 March). He suggested on 26 March that we hire Necropolis, 'and of course their pathologist Dr. Young.' I had been down this road before – with CDC. I called John and explained that we had an excellent pathologist in Charles Smith. And, most important, safety was Charles's number one concern.

Atlanta Workshop, April 1997

I arrived in Atlanta airport after 9:00 a.m. on 8 April 1997. I had told CDC that I was not available until 10:30 a.m. The meeting had begun at 9:30 a.m. I was very worried, as my team might have already decided to abandon the project after five years of my preparatory work. When I arrived at the institute, the meeting was in full swing. I knocked at the door, entered, and sat down beside one of the two men whom I had not met – namely, Lars Haaheim. The other stranger was Dr Jeffrey Taubenberger, whom I recognized from his photo in the newspaper. He was at the other end of the table. Unfortunately, I couldn't talk to him from where I sat.

At the first break, I walked over to Taubenberger and introduced myself. I apologized for missing his talk, the first of the morning, and explained that I could not fly in until that morning. I said that I was anxious to hear about his work. He replied, 'I thought you'd hate me because I beat you to it.'

'No,' I said. 'What you've accomplished is amazing.'

He offered, 'Perhaps we could meet later for drinks and discuss our research.'

'I'd really like that.'

But our conversation was cut short when Charles Smith came up to speak to me. 'Kirsty, it's fine. They want to go ahead with Spitsbergen.' I couldn't believe it. I thought the project was dead for sure. Next, Peter Lewin came over and gave me a hug, 'It's going very well, very well, indeed.'

The break was over. Lars Haaheim briefly described Norway's perspective on the project. Then I updated everyone present. I started with the most important news: the archival samples found by Daniel Perl and John Oxford's offer of archival samples. I then asked about the promised telephone hook-up to Daniel Perl in Guam and his promised samples. Brain Mahy said that the hook-up was not possible.

Mahy and Nancy Cox then informed us that CDC was no longer interested in archival samples. 'This project,' I protested, 'was to include both autopsy and archival material, as this was the consensus view among those present at the first workshop. Daniel Perl found both influenza and encephalitis samples following the discussion of our workshop.'[2] I was becoming accustomed to CDC's complete reversals of decisions. I was unprepared, however, when John Oxford began arguing against archival samples, some of which he had promised me in order to join my team.

CDC's change of heart clearly dumbfounded Rob Webster: 'I thought we all agreed to look at both types of material.,' he argued.[2] It was then suggested that Daniel Perl be dropped from the team because CDC no longer wanted archival samples. I countered, 'That's not fair.' But Nancy added, 'It's okay. Don't worry about Daniel. There's a man at Mount Sinai that he is very keen to work with.' The team didn't know, however, as I did, that Daniel planned to meet with Nancy the following week to discuss archival material.

After a heated discussion, a consensus emerged that the Spitsbergen project would deal solely with autopsy material. Only Rob Webster and I argued in favour of archival samples as well.

Alan Heginbottom gave a lengthy presentation regarding a site survey with ground-penetrating radar (GPR), which can be conceptualized as sonar for the ground. He explained that the radar would show the form of the original grave excavations. He estimated that a GPR study would cost Can.$20,000–25,000. Mahy said that CDC could provide up to U.S.$20,000, or more than enough to cover the estimated cost. Alan discussed the site excavation, which would be labour-intensive, since we could not use vehicles in the cemetery.[2]

John Oxford next gave a brief talk about Necropolis, a commercial company established after the Second World War to exhume the bodies of U.S. airmen. The company performs about 30,000 exhumations per year. Necropolis had particular experience with infectious corpses, such as smallpox victims. John was 'very keen' on Necropolis, as the 'company perceived that there was no risk in the exhumations.' He continued: 'Necropolis thought that the "real" risks are minimal and the "perceived" risks are the problem.' John pointed out that the company had no experience in working with frozen ground or with sampling frozen tissue. Charles Smith explained, 'Frozen bodies present more of a risk than unfrozen bodies.'[2]

Placing a body in ice is akin to storing it in a freezer. A freezer perfectly preserves food, and does not allow for decomposition. Because ice preserves, anthropologists have eaten, without adverse health effects, tissue from a mammoth entombed in glacial ice for 10,000 years. Placing a body in ice might therefore perfectly preserve a corpse and whatever killed the person. More to the point, burying a Spanish flu victim in the permafrost might preserve the body and the virus. Charles was disturbed by John's suggestion of no possible risk of infection, and particularly by slides showing an exhumation of a smallpox victim by an open window, near playing children.

The team agreed that only those essential should participate in the exhumations. At least two parallel sets of samples would be taken in stainless-steel tubes – just as we agreed at Windsor. We further agreed that John Oxford would approach the 'three big pharmaceutical companies which make anti-viral drugs' – namely, Ceiba-Geigy, Glaxo, and Roche, regarding funding. We stressed to John that any money accepted must have no strings attached. Robert Webster also agreed to look for funding on behalf of the team. Finally, we agreed that I would handle all funds through my university.[2] This was, symbolically and practically, extremely important. In academe, as in business, whoever has the money has the power.

The team's final order of business was to agree (by vote) to a scientific advisory group (SAG), consisting of Nancy Cox, Lars Haaheim, Alan Heginbottom, John Oxford, Robert Webster, and me.[2] I would have the expertise of the others to draw on, but my hands would be tied for virtually every decision from that day forward.

In closing, Brian Mahy announced that Peter Jahrling was to be a full-fledged team member.[2] CDC was appointing members to the team. But this time, I didn't argue. For over eight months I had wanted Jahrling as a member for his biosafety expertise, but I was concerned about his willingness to work with the Russians while committing himself to this project.

After the meeting adjourned, Brian led the team through the scientific wonders of CDC's BSL 4 laboratory. We viewed the full-body, pressurized 'space suits,' the laminar-flow biosafety cabinets, and the pass-through air-locks, which permit communication between the outer laboratory and the highest-containment area in the BSL 4 laboratory. The tour was informative.

Immediately afterwards, Jeff Taubenberger and I returned to our hotel for drinks. Jeff spoke first. He explained that the American Forces Institute of Pathology (AFIP) had been collecting tissue samples since the Civil War and that it has approximately three million cases. The fixed-tissue archives contain autopsy material from more than 100 victims of the 1918 influenza. One of those victims had fragments of the virus. Jeff's find was recognized as one of the top 100 science stories of 1997 (the same year as the cloning of 'Dolly' the sheep).

Jeff then told me of his difficulties in publishing his results and that he felt marginalized by the 'Influenza Mafia.' Jeff said, 'I don't trust them. I don't trust any of them.'

'Whom?' I asked.

'Virtually everyone sitting around the table this afternoon.' Jeff said, 'I don't know what Cox wants from me. But she wants something. I can't read her at all.' He continued, 'And Webster, he has been classy after the fact.'

He continued bitterly, 'Once I had results, I e-mailed *Nature* and asked whether or not they were interested in my paper. The answer was yes. One or two days later they rejected the paper. And a day after my rejection, the Mill Hill group [of which Dr Rod Daniels, the scientist I had met in Britain along with John Oxford, was an employee] asked for my samples.'

'That's unbelievable,' I gasped.

'I am convinced that *Nature* told the Mill Hill group about my work because there wasn't time for the paper to be reviewed by referees.'

Jeff had then applied to the other giant of academic publishing, *Science*. And within a few days, it too had rejected his paper.

'Finally, a guy who heard me lecture became my champion. At his urging, I sent the paper to Brian Mahy's journal. The first thing Mahy said to me at the conference today is that he was sorry he couldn't publish it. I bet he was.'

Then it was my turn. I told him of the history of the project to date. We commiserated about the difficulties of being young in academe/research, of not being a virologist in a 'virology' project. Jeff was chief of the Division of Molecular Pathology in the AFIP's Department of Cellular Pathology. I then invited him to be a member of our research team, as my team was very interested in having him participate. He said, 'Okay, boss. Friends.,' and we shook hands on the deal.

On 10 April, I wrote Jeff 'to extend a welcome to you and your family to stay with us in Toronto' for his upcoming conference. I heard back on the 14th: 'I wanted to let you know what a pleasure it was for me to have met you last week ... Let me know what else I can do to help ... Thanks for your interest in my music. I will shortly send you a tape of some pieces and the score for the two-part invention for piano.'

Jeff wrote me on 21 April, 'I am ... enclosing a tape of some of my music pieces and the score for the two-part inventions for piano ... Please let me know what you think, feel free to be honest! ... Thanks for your support.'

Aftermath: No Samples?

Following Atlanta, the team no longer actively pursued archival tissue samples. However, I wanted answers regarding formalin-preserved samples. I faxed Nancy Cox on 12 April: 'At the first workshop ... a total of 8 of the 10 team members ... wanted to pursue archival material. At our second workshop, I was surprised to learn that the team no longer wanted to examine archival material ... Only Robert Webster and I thought that we should examine archival material.'

I continued. 'Did Daniel Perl meet with you at CDC? What was the outcome of the meeting? Daniel Perl, a member of my project, and I (via John Oxford) had access to two archival data sets. Why is there now no interest in archival material? Why did you plan to meet with Daniel if there is no interest in archival material? Why wasn't John Oxford's offer discussed at the second workshop? Why is archival material not being included in the project when archival material is clearly being discussed/actively being pursued?' There was never any response to my letter.

I had invited Daniel Perl to join my team. He had found archival samples and had promised them to the team. However, he never turned over the samples.

A year after the meeting, Charles Smith was visiting CDC on non-flu business. He casually asked his colleagues if Nancy and Daniel had found fragments of the 1918 virus from their samples of archival tissue. He was informed that they had not.

The team never formally excluded Daniel. He simply drifted away.

And John Oxford? Despite his original promise, he never handed over his samples to our team. He would argue that the team decided on 8 April 1997 at CDC that it did not want archival samples. But a month after the CDC meeting, John wrote, 'I don't think you should worry about archive material. My offer is still open about sharing ours. We should concentrate on the Spitsbergen affair.' Regardless, I made good on my promise to make him a member of my research team. Obviously he should have honoured his personal promise.

After the CDC meeting, Nancy Cox wanted to talk to Dr McKee of the University of Iowa expedition to Alaska. At the meeting, I had referred to McKee as 'my source,' as I did not want to make trouble for him. Shortly afterwards, Nancy faxed me: 'I would be very happy to speak with your contact about the first exhumation of victims of Spanish influenza. I promise not to cause problems or be difficult about things when I call. Please go ahead and ask if he would be willing to speak with me. It would be good to get a better understanding of what laboratory tests were performed at that time, and very easy for me to ask the appropriate questions.'

I faxed Nancy on 9 May 1997: 'I just spoke with Dr. Albert McKee (my source), former University of Iowa virologist, who searched for the 1918 influenza virus in Alaska ... I asked if he would allow me to pass his name and number to you. I further explained that the team did not want to make problems for him, as he was quite worried about "problems" in our discussion.' I gave Nancy his phone number. Cox and McKee later arranged a telephone session. 'The conversation,' however, 'did not amount to much,' according to Nancy. (The secrecy regarding Dr McKee's identity and the need to protect his reputation seem more than ironic now, as I have since seen him interviewed at length on a documentary regarding his Alaskan expedition. It appears that he is no longer concerned about the lack of safety measures.)

Rob Webster faxed me on 15 April 1997, 'A window of opportunity is available for a small grant to the National Institutes of Health (NIH) that would support at least part of this study ... I am going to do my very best to submit an application at this time and would greatly appreciate your assistance by providing ... a letter of collaboration.'

I faxed back six days later: 'This letter is to confirm your collaboration with the project, "The identification of the 1918 influenza." On 22 April, Rob faxed me 'a rough draft of an application that is to be submitted to NIH before May 1 ... I would like to ask that you ... act as a highly critical reviewer.' On reading his application, I was so angry that I couldn't speak, I couldn't respond. Rob had made himself principal investigator on the project that I had conceived.

Both Charles Smith and John Oxford called me to see what I thought of Rob's proposal. Both men spoke, without my solicitation, to Rob on my behalf. John faxed me: 'I asked him to put you as Co-Principal investigator and to split the proceeds to your two institutions respectively [Rob's and mine] ... I put it very politely to him. He is a nice bloke basically.'

As a result, Rob called me on 22 April and assured me that he was 'not trying to cut you out.' I remembered his words from Windsor, 'None of us want to take what you've achieved.' And on 23 April, I faxed Rob, 'I am extremely pleased to accept the position of Co-Principal Investigator. Thank you for recognizing my work.' On 30 April, Rob faxed the team regarding the NIH grant: 'I especially want to acknowledge Kirsty Duncan's contribution to this project and it is appropriate that she be recognized as Director and Co-Principal Investigator.'

In May, John Oxford faxed me as well. 'You will be co-investigator with me as regards Roche and co-signatory on the cheques.' He faxed me each time he spoke with Roche – one of the world's leading healthcare companies and one of the most important in Europe – and gave me the good news regarding funding – a first offer of £20,000, and then a second of £25,000.

I responded with heartfelt thanks. On 22 June, John recommended that I 'have help ... for administration and coordinating the project. ' I had to that date spent over $23,000 of my own money on telephone calls, faxes, conference proceedings, mailings, and travel. I had previously applied for funding from the University of Windsor and from the National Geographic Society but had been turned down. I therefore had to pay expenses if I wanted the project to continue – although the university helped with expenses when it could.

Memorandum of Understanding (MOU)

As the project progressed, the need for a memorandum of understanding (MOU) became greater and greater if we were to ensure that all involved would receive their due credit and to prevent future academic squabbles. The University of Windsor had promised to write the MOU for me following the team's first workshop in August 1996. However, it produced no document, as the administration was tied up in negotiations.

As a result, I drafted a first version for the team's CDC meeting of 8 April 1997. On 24 April, I produced another draft following comment by the scientists. A day later John faxed me: 'I do think we have an excellent team of trustworthy people which you can depend on. If you are still worried about infection I could get Dr. G Lloyd the Lassa/Ebola expert to provide an independent assessment.'

John faxed me on 5 May, 'Overall the SAG of 6 which we have is most balanced (2 U.S.A., 2 Canada, 2 Europe).' At the time, I did not think about nationalities. Later, however, it would become apparent that the various countries voted en bloc. Science appeared to be similar to figure skating!

By 6 May the team was no further ahead with respect to the MOU, and this time John Oxford took a crack at producing one. A day later I met with the university lawyers to discuss the latest version and a contract that I had finally received from Associated Producers, which had filmed the Windsor Workshop. The lawyers thought the contract laughable – 'impossibly one-sided'! Associated Producers wanted me to sign my life away.

Duncan shall, at producer's request, disclose to Producer and Producer's representatives, subject to reasonable restrictions all information in Duncan's possession or under Duncan's control relating to the Expedition, including, without limitation, copies of any newspaper or magazine clippings, photographs, transcripts, notes, recordings, or other physical materials relating to the Expedition and Duncan's thoughts, observations, recollections, opinions, reactions, and experiences surrounding, arising out of, and concerning all those events, circumstances, and activities relating to the Expedition ... Duncan hereby grants, conveys and assigns exclusively and irrevocably to Producer, throughout the universe and in perpetuity, the right to depict the Expedition and Duncan and to use Duncan's name, image, voice and likeness ... Duncan hereby grants to Producer an exclusive thirty (30) day right of first negotiation and a ten (10) day right of last match with respect to the dramatic rights (television and feature film) in and to the Expedition and Duncan's life story in relation thereto.

I also discussed the MOU with the university lawyers.

In rewriting the MOU, I needed some pressing questions answered and verification of promises. I first faxed Dr Harvey Artsob of Health Canada on 24 April, and invited his involvement in the project. I hoped that Canada's BSL 4 laboratory in Winnipeg would be operational in time to analyse any samples retrieved from Svalbard.

I wrote to Nancy Cox on 12 May, 'I would like written verification that this team is not pursuing viable virus and that this team will undertake every safety precaution to prevent obtaining viable virus. The aim of this project has always been to sequence the 1918 influenza virus and not to obtain viable virus ... As Robert Webster wrote in his grant application, "although unlikely, the possibility must be considered of isolating the infectious virus."'

The question of infectious virus was crucial. Lars had offered to draft a letter to the Norwegian authorities, which I would sign, to request that the project be undertaken in two phases: a ground penetrating radar (GPR) study, and the actual exhumations, if warranted by the radar study. Lars insisted on writing that the team was looking for live virus. I repeatedly explained that recovery of live virus was never the aim of the project. Lars and I last spoke on 13 June. He insisted on live virus. And I refused.

John, CDC, and I, prepared repeated drafts of the MOU, and there was little agreement within the team. The MOU was threatening to tear us apart. On 12 June, John faxed me. 'I have had a fax from Lars. He seems to be in a slight lather about the MOU so I have suggested to him that he should treat it more lightly. It is after all a spirit document rather than a legal agreement. ' On the 23rd, John once again faxed me regarding Lars. 'I suspect some eruption from Lars! He has a bee in his bonnet at the moment. He will probably settle down when he returns to Bergen and gets off his high horse.'

CDC Withdraws

CDC's Brian Mahy faxed me on 17 June 1997: 'Unfortunately my budget at CDC is not good this fiscal year ... and we would not be able to make funds available for the September trip to Svalbard.' Two months earlier, at the CDC meeting, Brian had said that he could cover the costs of a radar study. CDC had changed its mind again.

And again. On 27 June, CDC faxed me: 'In view of the recent advances in sequencing the 1918 influenza genes, ... the urgency and novelty of exhuming the cadavers in Longyearbyen is not so apparent as it was when the project was first formulated. It is possible that other scientific groups in pathology and influenza virology will be spurred on by their success and will publish new findings using similar sources of archival material. Unfortunately, we are sorry that we cannot allocate the necessary time, effort and resources that the project now seems to require of us. It clearly deserves fully dedicated members in order to succeed. We therefore feel it is appropriate and for the benefit of the project that we step down, both as members of the Scientific Advisory Group and the team.' So Nancy Arden, Nancy Cox, Lars Haaheim, and Brian Mahy had all stepped down.

Just two months earlier, at the meeting in Atlanta, and despite Jeffrey Taubenberger's findings, they had agreed that the project should continue. Brian had initially promised funding for the GPR study. If 'the urgency and novelty of exhuming the cadavers in Longyearbyen' were no longer so apparent, that did not deter the man responsible for the 'recent advances.' Taubenberger confirmed his collaboration with the team on the grant application to the NIH. But since CDC had departed, I needed another BSL 4 laboratory. CDC's withdrawal could jeopardize the project's funding. And I needed a Norwegian co-ordinator. I had to act quickly.

Part Two

Ground-Penetrating Radar

6 New Members and GPR Preparations

June – October 1997

Three days after CDC withdrew on 27 June 1997, I faxed the Norwegian authorities: 'Plans for Phase 1 GPR analysis are progressing very well ... I would like to assure you that: (1) we have an excellent team; and (2) we are very keen to proceed with the project.' On the same day, I also faxed formal thank-yous to Haaheim, Arden, Cox, and Mahy 'for their time, effort, and work.' Meanwhile, John Oxford had written 'to ask them (Lars and CDC) to reconsider or, alternatively, suggest another Norwegian.'

Rob Webster was concerned that CDC's withdrawal might jeopardize our joint grant from the National Institutes of Health (NIH), and he wanted 'a big gun' to replace CDC's virologists. He asked about adding to the team Sir John Skehel, director of the National Institute for Medical Research (NIMR) in Mill Hill, London, previously director of the WHO's World Influenza Centre.

On 1 July I formally invited Sir John to join the team, and he consented the next day.

On 1 July, I received a phone call from our newest team member, Jeffrey Taubenberger, after he received my fax notifying the team that CDC had withdrawn from the project. Jeff asked, 'What's really going on with CDC?' I explained that Nancy Cox had planned to meet with Daniel Perl regarding found archival samples the week after our team's meeting at CDC. Jeff offered to 'try and get some information from Cox. I don't think I'll be able to though. Her answer to any of my questions is always "stuff,"' meaning that she did not divulge information.

Jeff, like Sir John, was on board. Because Lars Haaheim had withdrawn, we needed a new Norwegian co-ordinator, preferably a microbiologist/virologist, as Norway had suggested. John Oxford suggested Professor Tom Bergan, a friend of a friend, but highly recommended. Bergan had served as a professor at the University of Oslo since 1975 and was a consultant for the university's Institute of Medical Microbiology and the National Hospital. He was also the President of the International Society of Chemotherapy – a 20,000-member body concerned with both infections and cancer.

At John's suggestion, I wrote to Bergan on 10 July and invited him to join the project. After returning from holiday, he accepted my invitation on 27 August, and immediately provided information on Svalbard and even flight schedules for the upcoming GPR study.

Right from the beginning, I talked to or faxed Tom Bergan almost daily. I finally met him when he visited Toronto for a conference in late September 1997. After I guided him around Toronto's attractions, Charles Smith and I took him to dinner to discuss the science of our project and plans for the GPR study and the exhumations. We would be meeting him again in less than two weeks for the radar study, and he needed a good understanding of what had been planned.

John Oxford still worried that his friend Lars might make trouble for the team. On 7 July John faxed me: 'I am a little concerned that Lars might busy himself by making negative comments and so we should act quickly to get the Norwegian side in place (i.e. "get the Norwegians on our side").' I had, however, already spoken to and faxed the Norwegian authorities on 30 June to say that, even though CDC and Lars had pulled out, we had an excellent team.

Funding from Roche and NIH

I searched for funding for the GPR study. At the CDC meeting, Rob Webster and John Oxford had promised to try to secure funding – Rob, from NIH, and John, from pharmaceutical companies. Rob and I had a joint application at NIH, and John and I at Roche. On 10 July John and I had a commitment for £25,000 from Roche pharmaceuticals for Phase 1, the GPR study, more than the estimated cost for a four-person GPR team's travel and accommodation. John informed Jeff of the funding news, and on 5 August, Jeff faxed John: 'My wife and I just had a baby girl. Good news about Roche funding for Spitsbergen. Please keep me informed. Odd news about CDC pulling out of the project. Nancy seems to intimate that they are only interested in archival case material now. Do they have cases? Do you know if Robert Webster is still involved? What plans have been made for a new BSL 4 facility?' His archival search continued. 'We have been through about fifty [samples] with about 20 as yet unexamined. Are you looking only at lung or also brain? We have made good progress sequencing on our case. I have taken the last month to concentrate on ways to immortalize the RNA present for future analyses.' I immediately wrote to Jeff to congratulate him on the birth of his daughter and learned from him that 'Nancy Cox was concentrating on archival samples.'

I faxed Rob Webster on 11 August: 'Heartiest congratulations! Thank you for working so hard to win this formidable grant for the whole team ... Thank you for your excellent application to NIH and your extensive work and effort ... I know it was your name and fame that turned the trick!'

I couldn't believe it! The project was really going to take place. We had a promise of money from Roche and from NIH for the GPR study, which was less than two months away. I received more good news from John on 19 August. 'Roche has increased the grant to £30,000, payable within the next 30 days ... They have agreed almost certainly for the next year's budget of £100,000. Roche would like to handle media and have an international PR company to help. Their Toronto office will contact you directly. They would appreciate that one of their scientists join the team as an "associate member" (Dr. Noel Roberts).' I didn't like Roche's conditions. John had promised funding with 'no strings attached.'

More unsettling news followed on 1 September, with a copy of Roche's letter to John, 'As we discussed we are offering sponsorship on the understanding that we will be the only pharmaceutical company involved and that we have access to the proposed publications prior to their submission or release. As we agreed, this is not an attempt to alter or influence data or publication in any way, but to ensure that Roche and our affiliate organisations are aware prior to publication of what will be said about the project and, if appropriate, GS 4104 (the company's new drug).' Roche also wanted 'to offer professional assistance and help in the preparation, presentation and publication of activities and results from the subsequent investigations to ensure the maximum benefit to the project. I would strongly recommend the use of Hill & Knowlton (a public relations and public affairs consultancy).' As well, 'we would like to have a virologist on your committee to represent the interests of Hoffman La Roche. I would suggest Noel Roberts.'

The letterhead, address, and sender's name were omitted in the copy sent to me. Also, the letter was addressed to only John, despite our joint application. Confirmation of our status as co–principal investigators never arrived, despite John's numerous promises over the next few years; and the University of Windsor never received half of the grant money, as promised.

A conference call on 11 September among members of the SAG questioned Roche's involvement. Many members were concerned about the exclusive relationship. Rob Webster requested that John, 'go back to Roche and ask for non-exclusive rights, and no PR company.' However, we agreed, as a concession, to appoint Noel Roberts as a non-voting associate member.

I assume that Roche accepted John's requirements, because he later faxed me, 'Cheque has arrived! My interpretation is that this is "no strings" and £110K is further budgeted (for Phase ll, the exhumations). (I have the cheque in my hand.)'

No Memorandum, August–September 1997

The project was gradually coming together. Sir John Skehel had joined the team. We had a new Norwegian co-ordinator, Tom Bergan, and we had the all-important funding. Now, if we could only hammer out an acceptable agreement among the scientists.

After the University of Windsor failed to deliver the promised MOU, and after the team's bitter wrangling over repeated drafts throughout the spring of 1997, Rob Webster in frustration on 6 August, approached his institution, St Jude, in Memphis, to prepare an MOU. Yet the draft from St Jude required that American law govern my Ontario-born and Ontario-led project. I wanted the project to stay Canadian.

I could not operate under the regulations outlined in the document. If the University of Windsor was going to sign, I would simply have to quit my job. If I quit, no institution could sign the document on my behalf. On 14 August, I approached my other employer, the University of Toronto, for some help. I met with one of the vice-presidents, who provided excellent guidance.

Early the next morning, I called my department head and mentor, Professor Alan Trenhaile, and explained that I had to leave my job. I hoped that he would understand. I explained that I wanted to inform him of my decision before I told the university. Alan, always supportive and helpful, said that he would try to get the university to co-operate.

I soon called the vice-president, Dr Julian Cattaneo, to terminate my contract. An assistant took the call. I heard her say, 'It's Kirsty.' I then heard Julian in the background: 'Tell her I'm not here. I'm not taking her call.' Alan must have spoken to him before I had the chance.

Later that morning, Julian called me. 'Kirsty, we want to do whatever you want. The lawyers will be on it today.They'll do the MOU.' It was a little late. My American colleague had produced a document naming his workplace as lead institution! However, I agreed to give the university one last chance.

I later faxed Windsor, 'My chief concern regarding the agreement is that the project will be governed by the laws of Tennessee and that St Jude is the lead institution. My second concern is that I have lost power. Therefore, many of my comments relate to winning back power ... I appreciate that the other institutions may not like my comments. However, I need a workable agreement, within which I can operate and get the project done ... I walk a very narrow line; that is, I must keep control without upsetting my needed and valued team members.' I attached fifty-three amendments to the St Jude agreement. For example, I requested that 'the University of Windsor be the lead institution, as Duncan, the project leader, is employed by the University of Windsor'. I also asked that 'Duncan, as project leader, must come above the "Principal Investigators" (meaning that the project leader have authority over the SAG), as Duncan conceived the project, initiated the project, undertook all the background research and received the necessary permissions from the Norwegian authorities.' I further asked that 'the term "Principal Investigators" must not be used, and should be replaced by project leader and the scientific advisory group,' as 'the names of the six "Principal Investigators" do not correspond with the Co–Principal Investigators on the grant applications; the term "Principal Investigators" implies more prestige and honour than is granted'; and these were the terms agreed to by the team. I also asked why only the SAG institutions were to sign the agreement, and what would bind the remaining team members to the project?

While I communicated with Windsor, I received a fax from Rob Webster on 27 August indicating that, unless I signed his agreement, St Jude would not release the GPR funding. Rob warned, 'Let me reiterate that I believe it is a necessary precondition for St. Jude's ... participation that the Interinstitutional Agreement be signed by all parties before commencement of the project. St Jude's will not be able to release funds received from NIH for this study until this condition has been met.' Rob would not have been able to apply pressure if the NIH grant had gone to my university, as we agreed at the 8 April CDC meeting. But Rob's institution was to get the money, and it would therefore have the power. If Rob or St Jude did not like some aspect of the project, all he had to say was 'no money.' It was a powerful bargaining tool. However, I held the trump card – permission from the Norwegian authorities – and without me, they could not undertake the exhumations.

Rob continued to apply pressure, faxing me on 8 September: 'NIH has informed me that the Award Statement should be issued in the next few days. After the receipt of the award, St Jude Children's Hospital will be in a position to fund the project in accordance with the designated budget ... not yet received communication from the University of Windsor ... It is important that we get all of the formalities completed before September 11.' Windsor responded to St Jude on 18 September with my four pages of changes. On 24 September I passed on Tom Bergan's concerns to St Jude and asked for his support regarding my two chief requests: '(1) that the project stay Canadian-led and be governed by Canadian law; and (2) that the project leader description come above the description of the SAG (meaning that the project leader have authority over the SAG) ... Dr. Conta (St Jude) said that she would contact the members of the SAG regarding my two concerns. I would be grateful if you could support me.' I then called Alan Heginbottom and John Oxford to ask for their support. And on 25 September, Tom faxed St Jude: 'Dr. Duncan has mentioned two points which seem fair: 1, that the project stay Canadian-led, and 2, that the project leader be mentioned before the description of the SAG.'

I faxed Rob Webster: 'I am wondering if the Award Statement has been issued yet. Moreover, I am wondering if the grant money has arrived at St Jude ... I would be grateful if the money could be paid to the travel agent, as we are leaving (for the [GPR] study) in less than 2 weeks.' I was not going to sign the agreement if St Jude did not yet have the award statement or, more important, the money.

St Jude replied on the 26th: 'I have investigated your request for a revision to the Interinstitutional Agreement that the governing law be changed from U.S. to Canada. The Director of Research Administration at St Jude has provided the following information. The U.S. government requires that any research program which is supported by U.S. federal funds must be governed by U.S. federal law and policies, or by the laws of the grant recipient's state, whichever is more restrictive.

Thus, since the recipient of the NIH grant supporting the project ... is Webster/St Jude, the Agreement must designate U.S. law and Tennessee law.' My further questioning revealed that it didn't matter that I was the other recipient.

I was trapped. I needed to sign because of U.S. law and the required money. At the 8 April meeting, I was promised that all the grant money would go to my institution. However, this money would stay with Rob's hospital, and Roche's money would stay with John's institution. Their institutions would hold the purse strings. I regretfully signed the document on 2 October 1997.

Necropolis, July–October 1997

While I faxed St Jude to prevent the project's coming under American law, John Oxford began a campaign to involve the Necropolis Company, despite Charles Smith's concerns, mentioned above, about procedures proposed by Dr Susan Young, Necropolis's pathologist, for potentially infectious burials.

John Oxford on 10 July faxed me a copy of his correspondence to Rob Webster. 'Dr. Young was somewhat in favour of clipping the top half open and removing all internal organs for subsequent examination as in a "normal" type post mortem but I am not sure whether the Norwegians have agreed only to a small core sample.' John knew both that the team's first workshop had ruled out a 'normal' post-mortem because of potential risk of infection and that the Norwegians had agreed only to small core samples. Knowing that he would get nowhere with me, he got in touch with Rob Webster. Clearly, he did not appreciate that Rob's number-one concerns were safety and the protection of personnel and the environment. John would get nowhere with Rob.

On 12 September, John faxed me: 'I think that we must develop contingency plans for a 1997 exhumation immediately. ' Originally, I had wanted this too, but the American team hadn't prepared after the Windsor Workshop. We were undertaking the GPR study at the beginning of October. Polar night would soon follow and it would take months to analyse the GPR data and determine whether the exhumations were warranted. And most important, the safety precautions had not yet been fully planned.

John again faxed me: 'John Skehel is rather in favour of proceeding with the exhumations this year, but keeping it quiet from Lars. I have just spoken with Dr. Young. She is very positive ... and suggests that we proceed immediately in October.' John had earlier said on the phone, 'We have to do the work before Lars stops it!' Moreover, John was actively involving a non-team member, who was making suggestions regarding the operation of the project.

John would continue to solicit Young's opinions. On 11 September St Jude arranged a conference call for the SAG. John invited Dr Young to participate, and Rob Webster was outraged. It was a private meeting of the SAG. Even our team members other than the SAG were not involved. However justified, Rob's outburst was embarrassing to everyone on the phone, and so I sent a letter of apology to Dr Young, who did not join in the conversations.

On 3 October John ventured: 'Meanwhile we must plan quickly to exhume in December and hopefully achieve it before they all wake up. We could even work in Svalbard anonymously. It would have to be very quiet indeed.' I simply ignored the comments.

Preparing for Spitsbergen, August–October 1997

Who should travel to Longyearbyen? Originally, only a four-person GPR team – Alan Heginbottom, his assistant Les Davis, Charles Smith, and I – were to go. However, John Oxford repeatedly phoned and faxed me to include him. Since he was not part of the GPR team, he then suggested that the SAG should go. In addition, John recommended that Jeffrey Taubenberger be invited and asked him along.

John and Rob, who were holding the money, had spoken and decided that Jeff should go. 'Rob and I feel that the trip to the Arctic would be a carrot for Jeff to stay in our project. And we have the money.'

'But John,' I protested, 'I hold the grants with both of you.'

'The grant money is at our institutions. We sign the cheques.'

'John, you said that we would sign the cheques together. We would jointly approve all funding decisions.'

'Roche doesn't want that.'

I formally invited Jeffrey on 26 August.

Following my faxed invitation to Jeff, Jeff and I spoke on the phone. He wanted to go to Longyearbyen, and so I began making his arrangements. However, he soon informed me that he was 'extremely busy with the two babies and housing renovations.' He sent his regrets.

John and Rob talked privately and came up with a budget. The team would send the GPR group and the SAG. Rob Webster and John Skehel decided not to travel, but Sir John decided to send his employee Rod Daniels in his place.

John Skehel was making suggestions. Do I have another CDC on my hands? I wondered. Peter Lewin, involved from almost day one, was not going, but Rod Daniels was. I therefore requested money for Peter. I was told that there was no money and that a budget would not be forthcoming.

On 8 September, Tom Bergan, the team's Norwegian co-ordinator, agreed to travel to Longyearbyen. His long-time naval friend Professor Bjorn Berdal, director of Norway's Defence Microbiological Laboratory, volunteered to pay his own way. Norway's Directorate of Cultural Heritage determined that Berdal's lab should be involved in the project. In summary, the GPR brigade included: Bjorn Berdal, Tom Bergan, Rod Daniels, Les Davis, Kirsty Duncan, Alan Heginbottom, John Oxford, and Charles Smith.

In the weeks following, I made endless phone calls and reservations and sent numerous faxes. For almost a week, some 110 faxes came in daily from travel agents, airlines, hotels, and even clothiers. John Oxford, who had never been to the Arctic, thought that the team required a clothing allowance. I began phoning expedition clothing companies and faxing them information regarding the project. Would they sponsor us? The answer was always 'no.' In the end, John would allow each of us $500 for necessary clothing.

Flights were arranged. John informed me that his wife, Gillian, would accompany him to Longyearbyen. The rest of us were not bringing our spouses. The GPR expedition was a business trip, not a vacation.

I arranged accommodation, all meals, car, rental and transportation of the GPR equipment, carnets (custom permits), equipment insurance, health insurance, and meetings with the governor's office, the Directorate of Cultural Heritage, the church, and UNIS. Alan put together supply lists, and Tom Bergan arranged meetings with the health authorities.

I also checked if we should hold a short service prior to the GPR study and whether we could work on a Sunday if necessary. Pastor Hoifodt wrote that perhaps the team could attend a service at the church and speak to the congregation afterwards. It was, he said, acceptable for the team to work after the church service.

I inquired about polar bears, as a number of the team members were concerned. Should we bring flares or rifles? One team member took a course from the Royal Canadian Mounted Police on how to 'bring down a bear' were he to be attacked.

I also tried to hammer out a contract with Associated Producers. Since my university found the contract so one-sided, they recommended that I hire a private entertainment lawyer. There were numerous faxes throughout August and September. Heated negotiations continued until I finally told the lawyer on 25 September that the company could not film the GPR study. We simply could not come to an agreement. Meanwhile, John Oxford recommended that a British documentary company contact me, despite his knowing of my earlier commitment to AP.

While I arranged, booked, and negotiated, I also had to seek, as the SAG requested during our conference call, a second permission from the governor for exhumations in 1998 if the GPR study warranted them. I did not want to request permission, however, until after the study.

Although my waiting angered John, Tom Bergan understood my hesitation. Tom wrote to John on 13 September, 'I feel Kirsty is such a highly ethical person she feels that it would nearly be a lie if she submitted an application for 1998 now. She fears that Marstrander (Directorate of Cultural Heritage) might feel she has promised to base exhumation on GPR, but submitting an application now is consistent with that, since she only needs to state that there is not a plan to start digging before the GPR data have been processed.' Tom was right.

Tom thought that it was okay to ask for permission. He was Norwegian, and I would follow his lead. On 22 September I asked for a second permission. 'I appreciate that I am applying early for the permission (i.e. before Phase 1 GPR analyses); however, I believe that this is necessary in order to continue the project by properly planning ahead. I want to assure you, however, that the team will not proceed to phase ll if there is little evidence to suggest that the bodies of the seven miners are not well preserved.' I included Rob Webster's detailed protocol for Phase II, and a list of team members. I answered three questions that had appeared in the Norwegian press. First, the need to progress to Phase II in light of the work of Taubenberger et al.? Yes – confirmation, European data, unmodified material. Does the project pose any risk of infection? Absolutely minimal; rigorous precautions. Does the project pose any risk to the cemetery, a protected cultural site? Temporary scarring only.

I explained,

> There was a consensus among the team that the Svalbard permafrost material was needed in order to: (1) both confirm and extend the data from Dr. Taubenberger's group; (2) obtain virus from another location (in this case, Europe); and (3) obtain viral material that had not been chemically modified.
>
> Problems with the current data are as follows: (1) the information is incomplete (i.e. only 7% of the gene sequence has been identified); (2) the material studied has been exposed to formaldehyde, which is known to alter genetic material; and (3) the material studied has been stored at room temperature for 80 years and may be modified.
>
> It is significant and important that Dr. Jeffrey Taubenberger, who published the initial studies on molecular analysis of the 1918 influenza virus, has joined the project.
>
> A September, 1997, letter from Dr. Nancy Cox to Robert Webster includes the following: 'CDC supports the scientific merits of the project and I (Dr. Cox) will attempt to convey this to any members of the press who may contact me.'

Regarding the risk of infection, I continued:

> The possibility of obtaining infectious material is extremely low because: (1) the ground temperatures over the past eighty years have not been ideal for influenza viruses. The infectivity of influenza viruses is not stable for extended periods in the temperature range of –18° C to –4°C. At an assumed depth of burial of 1.0–1.5 m, the annual range of ground temperatures was not suitable for the virus. Viruses are conventionally stored at –70°C to maintain infectivity.
>
> Despite the extremely low risk, every safety precaution will be taken.
>
> It may be imperative to undertake the project for the following two additional reasons: (1) these bodies may, in the future, work their way to the surface ... The small possibility that these bodies may contain infectious virus warrants examination of the site to ensure biosecurity. (2) The existence of the bodies of the miners who died of the 1918 influenza is known internationally. This knowledge requires that a team with

the knowledge and the facilities to ensure biosecurity undertake the project.

Members of the team have consulted widely amongst colleagues. There has been considerable time to debate the benefits/risks of the project. If there had been concern from the health authorities or experts, the team would have been notified.

The team will use their considerable expertise to make sure that there is as little disturbance to the cemetery as possible. There will be a scar after the exhumation, as there would be with any interment, but expert opinion judges that the site will regain its original structure and appearance in time. The time would best be estimated by the Svalbard authorities who appreciate the extreme climatic conditions and slow growth in the Arctic.

On 24 September I faxed an addendum to my letter asking for permission. 'I asked Professor Lewkowicz (Associate Professor, Department of Geography, University of Ottawa) for his expert opinion regarding the feasibility of the project. Lewkowicz is a permafrost specialist and is not associated with the project.' Lewkowicz wrote: 'In summary, I believe that from the point of view of avoiding frost heave of the bodies and permafrost preservation, the project is feasible. With the precautions ... it should be able to be accomplished with minimal disturbance to the site.'

On 29 September 1997, a feature article, 'The Dead Zone,'[1] in the *New Yorker Magazine*, detailed the hunt for the 1918 influenza virus and described our project very favourably. I had asked a number of my team members, including John Oxford, if they would let reporter Malcolm Gladwell interview them. In the end, John was not interviewed, and when the article appeared he was very upset. He decided that he wanted both a media embargo and a public relations company to handle all media – clearly, a contradiction.

It was the end of September 1997, and we had no way of paying for the trip. St Jude had yet to receive the NIH grant money, despite earlier trying to force me to sign the MOU. And Rob Webster was reluctant to use John Oxford's money, because Rob could use the NIH money only for what the grant application specified – namely, a four-person GPR team. John was also reluctant to pay for the trip. He suggested that everyone pay for his or her flight and accommodation prior to departure. Alan was retired. I had spent over $23,000. Charles and Alan had already paid to travel to Windsor and Atlanta. I was tired of their paying. John would not cover the major costs (up front) but was willing to grant money for clothing.

On 25 September, the project was clearly in jeopardy. Alan had an idea that I faxed to John – Roche should pay all expenses, and the travel agent would then issue a second invoice to St Jude when its NIH grant arrived. I also explained how John could send me the money for my travel agent via Western Union. But John didn't think it possible to issue the cheque. His college would need more time to process the draft. However, John had had Roche's cheque for quite some time; Roche had authorized the invoice to be paid on 31 August 1997. On 30 September, I again faxed John. 'It would be wonderful if the College could release the funds tomorrow and the money could be sent via Western Union.'

Alan called the same day. 'Are we going?' he asked.

'I don't know. Things are down to the wire, and John doesn't seem concerned. He wants all of you to pay up front.'

'If he does, I'm not going, and there will damn well be no GPR study.'

'Alan, I don't want you to pay again. I promise that I won't let that happen.'

'What is the guy trying to do? Come in and be big hero at the last minute?'

Finally, on 2 October John sent the cheque to my travel agent via UPS. It was guaranteed for Saturday delivery. The cheque, however, did not arrive until Monday, and we left the next night, 7 October, for Longyearbyen.

7 Through the Ground Darkly

October 1997

I was off to Spitsbergen once more, along with Alan and Charles. Together, the three of us flew first to Frankfurt, then to Oslo, and finally to Longyearbyen. Sitting with my friends on the first two planes, I did not have time to contemplate what the next week would bring. However, alone in my Oslo hotel room, I allowed myself to think ahead. Would the radar show disturbance of the ground? Would it locate the miners' graves? If the answers were 'no,' my five-year project would end. Everything was riding on the GPR study.

I went to meet with John and Gillian Oxford, Rod Daniels, and Les Davis, Alan's Canadian GPR technician. John greeted me reservedly. He appeared to still be smarting from not being mentioned in the *New Yorker* article. Gillian confirmed what I had been thinking: 'My husband should have been mentioned in that *New Yorker* article you faxed over.' As an interviewee, I had no say over whom the journalist interviewed or what the finished article covered. I replied, 'I have been looking forward to meeting you.'

Gillian, together with John, next faced off against Les. 'You'll have to sign an agreement. Your company cannot sell any radar pictures to the papers. They'll be worth a lot of money.' Les was both offended and angered. Neither John nor his wife appreciated that the GPR would show nothing so specific as coffins or bodies – only disturbance of the soil.

Dinner went no better. Gillian first reminded us that her daughter Esther was a journalist and that John was used to being interviewed by documentary companies and newspapers. 'The media coverage is ever so important in this project. The team needs a spokesperson. John, you should do it.'

It was a long evening, followed by two equally long flights the next day: from Oslo to Tromso and from Tromso to Longyearbyen. Gillian, carrying John's two-foot-high, yellow, papier-maché model of an influenza virus, was interested in all things 'team' during the flights.

On landing in Tromso, we were surprised to meet Roger Webber, from the Necropolis Company, invited by John to Longyearbyen. The SAG should have had the opportunity to decide whether or not he was to be invited. I assume that John paid for Webber's flight, as John refused to answer any of my questions about the travel arrangements.

From the airport in Longyearbyen, the team was to take a car straight to the governor's office. As we loaded the van, I turned to Mrs Oxford and said, 'Gillian, Les will not be coming with us to the governor's office, as he is not a team member. He has however kindly offered to accompany you to the hotel.' I was trying to soften the blow to Gillian, who seemed to consider herself a team member. She would not be the only person left out.

'Yes, Gillian, I'll take you,' Les chimed in.

'Thanks, Les,' I said. Charles whispered, 'Nicely done.'

However, as we climbed out of the van, I heard Gillian talking loudly to her husband behind our vehicle. 'That woman, that woman, won't let me go to the governor's office. What are you going to do about it? I want to go, John.'

'Don't worry, love, you'll go. I'll see to it. You have to carry the virus.'

I called John aside. 'John, I'm sorry, but Gillian cannot come to the office. It is a private and requested team meeting.'

'Gillian is coming with me. She'll cause no trouble. I'll give her the virus to carry.'

'John, she can't come.'

'Kirsty, she is coming. Remember who is funding this study.'

The meeting was a fiasco. Gillian placed the large yellow virus in the middle of the table as both a centrepiece and a conversation stopper and was pleased when the vice-governor asked her what it was. She proudly announced, 'An influenza virus.'

I ignored her remark, said what an honour it was for all of us to be present in Longyearbyen, and quickly introduced the team. Gillian, who should not have been present, introduced herself. We all looked helplessly at John to quiet his wife, who had numerous questions for the governor's office, including, 'Can we exhume this year?'

Gillian then gave us her views on the media and the ethics of disturbing a cemetery. She even questioned why 'all this permission'

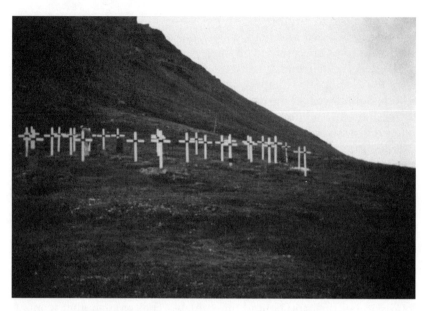

Figure 4   Longyearbyen cemetery.

was necessary. The Norwegians politely answered all her questions. I thought that the meeting would never end. I had spent two years developing a relationship with the office and convincing it that our project was serious, and Gillian had shared her toy virus.

Site and GPR Survey

The next day, Alan, Charles, and Les headed off to the cemetery (Figure 4) to begin the initial site survey, while I journeyed out to meet with Longyearbyen and to renew old friendships. Once again, it was necessary that I become part of the community, and not merely a foreign researcher. My first visits were to Mr Mork and Mr Holm, teachers at the local school, and Pastor Jan Hoifodt of Svalbard Kirke. Jan, on opening his door, said, 'Kirsty, you must have the team over. I will make caribou stew. I have been lucky hunting this year.'

I then walked to the cemetery to assist Alan, Les, and Charles, who had already begun the site survey and the GPR. A camera was rolling. Charles said, 'There's been some trouble. The camera crew is from Iceland. John has been very rude to them. It's okay though, I've talked to them.'

'What about Gillian?' I asked.

'She, too, has had things to say to the Icelandic crew.'

I walked over to Les. He was fit to be tied. 'Get them out of here,' he said under his breath.

'Who?'

'John and Gillian.'

'What's the trouble?'

'He keeps asking me what's happening. We haven't even started. I can't work with the two of them hovering over me.'

While Les and I spoke, Alan was carefully preparing a large-scale plan of the cemetery (located on a southeast-facing slope at an elevation of about 60 m) and the surrounding area. The plan (Figure 5) included the graves of the seven Spanish flu victims (at left in row 1, at top), all adjacent graves, all grave markers and fences, the access road, the entrance, and the adjacent public road. The survey would later allow us to plan spatial arrangement of the excavation, the order of the grave excavations, and the placement of the tent.

Alan next laid a grid over the highest three rows of graves, which rise 10 to 20 cm above the general level of the ground and are edged with fieldstones. Individual graves are marked with either white wooden crosses or gravestones. Most plots contain a single grave. However, two plots contain two markers, one has three, and one houses the seven markers of the Spanish flu victims.[1] Alan's grid would allow the four-person GPR team to guide the radar along the cemetery surface and record accurately what lay beneath the ground. As Alan hammered in stakes and strung flagging tape between poles, I remembered my July 1997 lesson in GPR with Les, Alan, and Charles at Canadian Forces Base Borden near Barrie, Ontario, where Les's company, Sensors and Software, had buried tanks and pipes for aiding instruction in GPR use.

The radar – in effect, sonar for the ground – has been used to locate murder victims, land mines, and even the Lost Squadron – six P-38F fighters and two B-17E Flying Fortresses buried 80 m deep in the Greenland Ice Sheet.[2] GPR employs radio waves to detect buried objects in any non-metallic material, such as soil, ice, rock, and human-made structures. It can penetrate depths from a few metres to many tens of metres depending on soil conditions. Low radio frequencies are used for deep exploration, and high radio frequencies for high-definition imaging.[3] A sensitive detector is dragged across the surface of the material under investigation. Radio waves are sent down through the material and are reflected from embedded objects. A computer

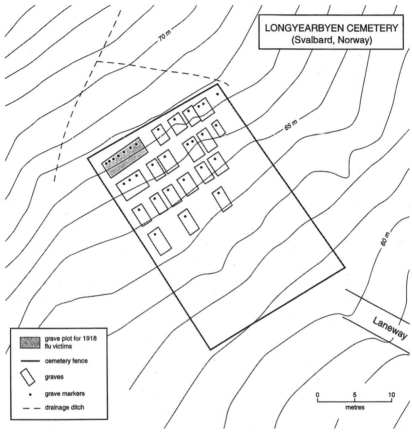

Figure 5   General plan of the cemetery (rows 1–4 of graves, from top).

records and merges the data to create images of vertical sections of the material under investigation.

I then watched while a leading geologist, geophysicist, and pathologist dragged the GPR equipment 100 times over the bumpy, frozen tundra and waited, with bated breath, while the images slowly materialized on the computer screen. What did the images mean? What was beneath the surface? Was it buried deeply? And was it frozen?

But John Oxford, who was demanding immediate answers from Les, did not seem to realize that it would take months for Les to analyse the megabytes of data. Les was quickly losing patience with John, and so the GPR technician gave Oxford a job to keep him busy. John was to hit a specific key of the computer whenever Les demanded 'F ... F ... F' of his over-zealous assistant.

Tom Bergan, his wife, Bodil, and Bjorn Berdal of Norway's Defence Microbiological Institute joined us in Longyearbyen that night. Bodil shared Norwegian stories, history, recipes, and chocolate with us and quietly supported her husband and the team.

During a lively party that Pastor Hoifodt gave, Tom and I cut a cake to launch the project. Our host told me of a family that had lost its teenage son a few years earlier, frozen to death just 200 metres from home. The family feared that the son's grave, which lay in the same row as the Spanish flu victims, would be disturbed. I asked Jan, 'Should I go to speak to the family?'

'No. Wait to see what they do.'

Shortly thereafter, the father came to the cemetery. Charles noticed him first and went over to speak to him. Charles then introduced the man to me, and I could see immediately that Charles had put him at ease. 'I am so sorry for your loss. And I am sorry that this project is hurtful to you and your family. I will do my best to make it right for all of you. In no way will we harm your son's grave.' The man politely acknowledged what I had said. I then added, 'I would be honoured if you would help me with the radar. Would you take the soundings with me?' He agreed. We each picked up an antenna, knelt on the ground, and began sampling.

I would remain in touch with the family. The mother later wrote to me in Canada and enclosed a beautiful picture of a young boy.

At Sunday service at Svalbard Kirke, a number of team members joined in 'Cantai ao Senhor um cantico novo' (Sing a new song to the Lord). We also enjoyed the psalms read in Norwegian and meeting townspeople, including a beautiful baby boy, whom I would meet again almost a year later.

John would periodically try to make amends: 'Gillian brought her dance shoes. Perhaps you and she can dance together.' I thought not. And Gillian herself was no longer interested in performing a reel or a jig, as she had taken to singing Irish airs for the team, and John, to reciting his own poetry.

After dinner, a few of us met in the hotel bar. A live band was playing Norwegian rock and roll, John and Gillian invited me to dance, and I asked Rod and Les to join us. John then began making digging movements and singing with gusto, 'Hi ho, Hi ho, it's off to dig I go.'

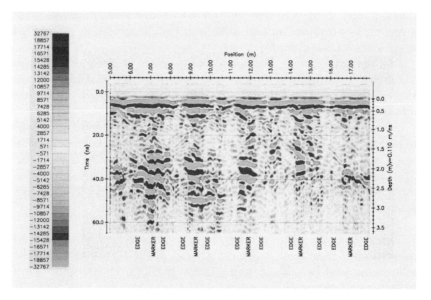

Figure 6   The GPR record over row 3 of the cemetery.

'John, stop that,' I exclaimed, appalled, and left for my hotel room.

The team managed to collect 100 profiles of the cemetery – each vary-ing in length from 8 m to 25 m. We sent radio waves down through the frozen ground every 2 cm along each of the 100 profiles. The huge quantity of data almost wiped out the hard drive of one computer.[4]

I met with all local parties interested in our work. We held an infor-mation meeting at UNIS for the people of Longyearbyen, who had consented to the project. First, I briefly described the project's history. Then Alan presented a slide (Figure 6) showing a GPR data plot from the third row of the cemetery. He first pointed to the horizontal axis of the plot, which shows distance in metres along the survey line. Alan explained that the markers or crosses and the edge of the graves appear on the horizontal axis. The geologist then highlighted the verti-cal axis which shows echo travel time and depth. Alan described initial results. The red and blue signals on the slide represented strong sig-nals, typically indicating disturbed ground. Red and blue signals cor-respond to markers, and few or no signals, to areas between grave markers. These colours would suggest that bodies/coffins might lie

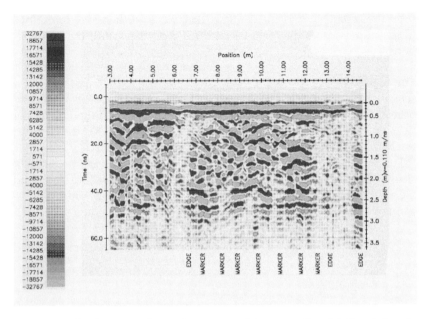

Figure 7   The GPR record over the graves of the seven Spanish flu victims (at left in row 1).

beneath the grave markers. Alan also explained that in some cases signals are shown without the presence of a marker on the surface – perhaps because of unusual rock formations.

Alan then presented a slide showing the GPR data plot of the graves of the seven Spanish flu victims. Excitedly, he pointed to a large disturbance corresponding to the seven graves, marked by six crosses and one headstone (Figure 7). He explained that something might lie beneath these markers. But that is all that Alan could say; he and Les would need months to interpret the data.

Charles spoke about his recent use of GPR in a multiple-murder investigation stretching from India to Canada. Rod explained in detail the structure of the influenza virus. And finally Tom talked in Norwegian about biosafety.

Following the meeting at UNIS and before Tom's departure for Oslo, our Norwegian co-ordinator arranged for a wreath to be laid at the cemetery and for *Svalbardposten* to record the event. We laid a wreath while the winds swirled around us, stirring up coal dust and debris from the cemetery, and the cameras flashed. And then I said goodbye to the miners, perhaps for the last time ... perhaps until the exhumations.

The meetings in Oslo went very well. We had earlier worked out a scheme to prevent any unwelcome questions. I would answer all questions at the Directorate of Cultural Heritage and would then turn over the floor to the most appropriate person. Tom would do the same at the Norwegian Ministry of Health.

Following the meetings, we all headed home. Phase I – the GPR study – had been a success.[5] We had collected megabytes of data, and we continued to work closely with the people of Longyearbyen. The team would now have to wait patiently to see what the data revealed.

Part Three

Wrestling with Demons

8 Live Virus?

October 1997–January 1998

A future trip to Longyearbyen would depend on the results of the team's GPR study. If the results showed disturbance beneath the markers of the seven influenza victims, and below the active layer of the permafrost, we would return to Norway. If the results did not meet these parameters, the project would cease. A month later, I was pleased to received an e-mail from Dr Alfred Crosby, whose 1976 book had inspired my search: 'I have heard a great deal about you and your Svalbard project from Dr Taubenberger and now "The New Yorker." I wish you luck, one, because you may find out something that will block the return of the 1918 bug, and two, because you have stimulated more interest in my book than anybody or anything ever.'

Invitation to the NIH, November 1997

Dr Dominick Iacuzio faxed me on 19 November 1997, to invite me to the National Institutes of Health (NIH) in Bethesda, Maryland, to discuss the project. 'This is an invitation for you to join a select group of individuals to participate in a one-day meeting to review the plans and progress of [your] scientific expedition to the town of Longyearbyen, Svalbard, Norway. The National Institute of Allergy and Infectious Diseases (NIAID) awarded an expanded international research supplement grant award to Dr Robert Webster to participate in the expedition to validate the nucleotide sequence of the influenza virus responsible for the 1918 pandemic.' Iacuzio called our project 'an important step in generating a better scientific understanding of the 1918 influenza strain which caused the most devastating pandemic in recorded history. Everyone will agree that the information gained from this expedition may help to prepare for a future pandemic. We recognize that there are risks associated with this project which involves the cooperation and resources of several Governments, agencies, and scientific institutions. In addition to representatives from NIAID, representatives from other governments and agencies have been invited.'

Our project was clearly being judged on its scientific merits, and its possible benefits were being recognized. Yet why was only Webster mentioned as recipient, rather than both of us? However, NIH was considering funding Phase II. Former project members Nancy Cox and Brian Mahy would now be among the experts deciding on funding, as would current members, Jeffrey Taubenberger and Peter Jahrling, who would of course support the project. I hoped that Jeff's partner, Ms Ann Reid, and his superior, Dr Timothy O'Leary, might also support the project, as well as Health Canada's Dr John Spika. (I was trying to arrange for any samples collected from Svalbard to be shipped to Canada. Two days before going to NIH I flew to visit Health Canada in Ottawa to meet with Dr Harvey Artsob and discuss involvement of Canada's BSL 4 laboratory.) I couldn't begin to guess how influenza greats Dr Edwin Kilbourne (New York Medical College) and Dr William Jordan (NIAID) would rule on the project.

A day after receiving Iacuzio's invitation to NIH, I received a fax from Jeff. He was withdrawing from the project. Astounded, I called him. He apologized. His boss had forced him to send the fax. He apologized again.

Jeff said that he heard that the team was going after live virus and that we had been charging for interviews. 'Jeff, none of that's true. You know that. Lars Haaheim wanted live virus. In fact, he wanted live virus recorded as a specific aim of the team in the MOU. I refused, saying that live virus was a risk of the project, and not an aim, as stated in the NIH grant application. And as for interviews, Jeff, you know the money that I'm out of pocket. How could you say that I was charging anything?'

'I'm sorry.'

'Jeff, I want you as part of my team. Would it help if I were to write to your boss to clear up the misunderstandings?'

'Yes.'

On 24 November, I faxed both Jeffrey and his boss, Dr Timothy O'Leary, explaining that the allegations in Jeff's letter were simply untrue. There was no response to either fax. However, I would be seeing Jeff in less than two weeks at NIH, and I was sure that the whole mess could be sorted out then.

Live Virus? NIH Meeting, December 1997

4 December 1997. I arrived first at NIH along with Nancy Cox. We made small talk, and she kindly asked me about the project's progress. When Jeff arrived, I went over to greet him and ask about his new daughter, Hannah, and his family. He showed me pictures of both his children and his recent home renovations. And then he said, 'Kirsty, it's okay. I can participate in the project.'

'Jeff, that's wonderful. I knew it could all be sorted out. None of what was written was true.' I guessed that O'Leary appreciated my letter. There was no more time to talk, as the meeting was starting. Jeff and I sat together – as he said, 'for moral support.'

The first order of business was Jeff's update on genetic information of the 1918 influenza virus. It was necessary for Jeff to update the expert panel on his latest findings so that everyone involved could make an informed decision as to whether or not there was a need for the Svalbard material.

Rob Webster later reported to Sir John Skehel: 'Jeffrey Taubenberger indicated that he now has the complete sequence of the hemagglutinin gene and was extremely cagey at this meeting and provided little or no input on the extent of sequencing of the other genes. He did indicate that he has three other positive samples for analysis. There seemed to be an underlying question of priority rights to this information and he was very nervous.'

When the group pushed Jeff to say whence his new positive samples came, he looked across the table to his boss, O'Leary, for help. I then understood why O'Leary sat where he did. O'Leary explained that they were not at liberty to share that information.

Rob Webster next presented options for obtaining additional information on the Spanish flu. As he spoke, I dashed off a note congratulating Jeff on his newest successes. Rob explained that fixed tissues from the United States and Europe might provide answers – I assumed that he meant the samples that Jeff, Daniel Perl, and John Oxford had. Rob further explained that samples of swine tissue might also provide clues. Regardless, there were very few samples, and more information was needed.

John Spika of Health Canada added, 'Even if you had twenty sequences from different places, you should still plan to dig.' Spika was on side. Edwin Kilbourne also appeared supportive, as he even suggested looking at burials through the 1920s.

And then Jeff spoke. Having told me before the meeting that he could participate in the project, Jeff now suggested to everyone present that the project should not go forward. Jeff had asked that we 'sit together for moral support.' When did he change his mind?

Rob Webster later wrote to Sir John: 'The group from the Armed Forces Institute of Pathology (Jeffrey Taubenberger's Institute) including Dr Timothy O'Leary, was extremely critical of the project; they do not believe that there would be any RNA of any length due to the temperature ranges in the permafrost over the years. I don't know why they can be so certain of this, especially if virus particles were present. They also questioned the temperature prior to burial and whether there is any possibility of RNA. They consider it a very long shot.'

I tried to recover from my initial shock. I had to present the background and history of the project and, more important, the results of the GPR study. 'The area of the gravesite of the seven Spanish flu victims has significant disturbance in the ground, suggesting that it is the location of a number of graves. The depth of the active layer of permafrost over the graves is 0.8 ± 0.2m (that is, the active layer lies somewhere between 0.6 m and 1.0 m). Based on air temperature records at Longyearbyen from 1910 to the present, it is likely that the active layer has never been deeper than one metre at this site. The GPR did not show coffins; however, it did show disturbed ground. The disturbance extends to 2 m in depth at all the grave areas surveyed in the cemetery, and thus it is likely that the coffins/bodies are at, or deeper than, 1.5 m. Therefore, it is likely that if material is beneath the surface, it has been frozen for the past 79 years. Based on the data, the team recommends continuing the planning for the exhumations.'[1]

Rob outlined the proposed exhumations, and detailed recommendations on biosecurity. Later he reported to Sir John: 'There was uniform consensus that the possibility of obtaining infectious virus was extraordinarily low but that biosecurity steps must include the possibility of infectious virus.' Kilbourne put the risk at 10^{-18}. Rob's communication to Sir John continued. 'A straw ballot at the end of the meeting indicated that 50% of those present would attempt to isolate the virus.'

The expert panel was discussing live virus. I interrupted. 'My project is not about live virus. Live virus has never been the aim. I just want to make that clear to you.'

The final agenda item concerned public and press considerations. After a lengthy discussion, Jeff accused me of charging for interviews. I then faced a barrage of questions from the scientists and the people from NIAID.

After the meeting adjourned, there was little time to talk, as I had a plane to catch. Jeff promised that he would be in touch with me shortly. I then looked for team member Peter Jahrling, whom I had never met. He was talking with a friend. I waited patiently for him to finish, but he did not wrap up his conversation. Eventually, I excused myself, 'Dr Jahrling, I'm Kirsty. I apologize for interrupting your conversation, but I have a plane to catch. I was wondering if you had a minute to talk.'

He dismissed me: 'I'm speaking, Ms. Duncan.' He had wanted to attend the Windsor Workshop but then backed out because of CDC. He provided me with information on Swords into Plowshares. He even joined my team. And when we finally had a chance to talk, he was 'speaking.'

There was one more person with whom I wanted to talk, Edwin Kilbourne, who soon came up to me and said, 'Kirsty, congratulations, it's a good project.' I was elated. One of the best-known flu men in the world liked the work.

A day after the meeting, I faxed Rob Webster: 'Thank you for your great effort on behalf of the project. I am truly grateful to you. Moreover, thank you for your kindness and your encouragement. It was wonderful to see you in action – you were both a scholar and a gentleman.

Jeff's Wavering

After my experience with Jeff at the NIH meeting, I decided to see if he was truly participating in the project. I faxed him on 20 December 1997: 'I would be most pleased if you are able to participate in the project. Would it be possible to fax me a list of what you need from the team in order to participate? Heartiest congratulations on your recent successes! Please pass along my congratulations to Ms. Reid' – she was one of Jeff's collaborators from the AFIP on the March 1997 paper in *Science* on characterization of the 1918 virus.

There was no response to my request until 13 January 1998, when Jeff informed me that he could not participate. When I called him, he explained that his institute was still concerned about live virus and charging for interviews. I replied, 'I thought I made it quite clear to all present at NIH that both allegations were untrue.'

'We need confirmation.'

I wondered how I could confirm that we weren't going for live virus – except to say precisely that – and that we weren't charging for interviews. Did I require signed notes from all interviewers?

I still believed, however, that Jeff's institution and our team could come to an agreement. I also believed that Jeff could make an invaluable contribution to our team; his team had been, after all, the only one to characterize genetically the 1918 Spanish influenza virus. And so on 15 January I faxed the SAG. 'Dr. Taubenberger is unable to participate in the project until his institute is convinced that a number of issues are addressed. Dr. Taubenberger is a valued member of our team. We must, therefore, work through the issues of concern.'

While Jeff wavered, the team elected two new full members – Bjorn Berdal and Les Davis. In addition, at Roche's request, it accepted Dr Noel Roberts as a non-voting associate member.

Meanwhile, the media were still a concern. On 18 November 1997, I received a fax from Simcha Jacobovici, Elliot Halpern's partner in Associated Producers. He was angry that the team had said no to their contract. 'At this time, we are hereby putting you and SAG on notice that we take the position that we already *have* an agreement with respect to this project and that we believe that you have acted in bad faith in your negotiations over the long form agreement and in the manner in which you have sought to break off those negotiations.'

I responded on 25 November: 'Perhaps you are unaware that Mr Halpern understood and agreed (in our telephone conversation of 14 August 1997) that any contract would have to be reviewed by the SAG (a six-member group), as directed by the team's Interinstitutional Agreement, a legal document signed by the institutions of the SAG members. I explained to Mr Halpern on 14 August 1997 (and indeed in following conversations) that the SAG would have the right to accept/ reject any contract. Mr Halpern accepted this state of affairs. My lawyer was made aware of this constraint verbally and in writing on 15 August 1997.'

Associated Producers finally produced a draft "Agreement" on 28 April 1997 (nine months after our initial meeting). The University's law firm reported on 12 August 1997: 'The Contract is extremely one-sided. Instead of trying to fix the contract by suggesting amendments, in our opinion, you would be better off by having a new contract drawn up which is consistent with your expectations.'

My letter continued. 'On September 29th, 1997, I explained to my lawyer that Associated Producers would be unable to film Phase I, as no (acceptable) contract had been provided.' Nevertheless, Halpern was in Copenhagen on 6 October, with a film crew on stand-by. 'On October 7th, 1997, I received the promised contract by fax at 2:53 p.m. I left for the airport to travel to Longyearbyen for the Phase I expedition at 2:55 p.m. ... Also, on October 7th, 1997, your Office contacted me at the airport (as I was boarding the plane!) to say that they were sending me, via courier, a copy of the contract ... On November 9th, 1997, I polled the SAG regarding the contract. In my letter of 13 November 1997, I did not include the disparaging comments of the scientists. Finally, as you point out in your letter, negotiations have been underway. If negotiations are underway, it is implicit that no agreement exists ... I think that you will agree that a documentary is now impossible, as there is mistrust on both sides.'

Having finished negotiations with Associated Producers, I was now free to follow the team's request that I negotiate with National Geographic. After meeting with the organization in Washington, DC, I faxed the SAG on 20 December: 'I sincerely hope that you will be pleased by National Geographic's interest, as both the magazine and television are world-renowned.'

Despite this, John Oxford faxed me on 12 January 1998: 'I met the CBS team, Horizon and Elliot from AP as well as the Garfield Kennedy Group. They seem to have formed a conglomerate, encouraged by the BBC Horizon team and will, I am sure, make some proposals about Svalbard 1918 ... I feel personally that it would be satisfactory if we could forget the previous "hitches" and start anew.'

On 6 January 1998, I received an e-mail from Dr Christopher Longyear, grandson of J.M. Longyear, a founder of the Arctic Coal Company on Spitsbergen in 1904. 'I am writing to ask for information about the project to exhume miners in Longyearbyen and for suggestions of how I might be an observer without inconveniencing those carrying out that important research. My motivations are both personal and professional ... My grandfather, John Monroe Longyear, was actively involved in exploring Spitsbergen, then developing the place still called Longyearbyen (or Longyear City) and its coal mine, which was owned mainly by Longyear and his partner, Frederick Ayers, from 1905 through most of 1916 ... My interest in the language of DNA and RNA has been further stimulated by the notice taken to recover the RNA of the pandemic influenza virus of 1918 from miners buried in the permafrost near Longyear City.'

I wasn't sure how to respond. We could have no observers. However, I did not want to put Longyear off, as he might be able to provide new information, and he was also a wonderful link with Svalbard's past. I thought that Norway should know about him. As a result, I consulted Tom Bergan. He suggested inviting Longyear to the team's next meeting, scheduled for 3 February 1998 at the NIMR.

I received a much-anticipated fax on 14 January from Lyder Marstrander of Norway's Directorate of Cultural Heritage: 'The Directorate is now prepared to make a decision about your application for the continuation of your project. Both the Science Council and the Health Service are positive. It would be very good if you could send me a letter stating whether you will continue or not.'

I responded on 19 January: 'I am thrilled that the Directorate is now prepared to make a decision regarding the project ... The field work yielded very positive results ... A field report, "Locating the Graves of Seven Spanish Flu Victims in Longyearbyen Cemetery, Svalbard, Using Ground Penetrating Radar" will be sent to you very shortly ... Continued planning for phase II will take place during the team's 3 February 1998 meeting at Mill Hill, London, England. I will send you a report following the meeting.'

Preparations for Mill Hill

John Oxford faxed me on 19 January: 'Hopefully if everyone would have the time I would like to invite the team to visit both St. Bartholomew's Hospital and the Royal London on February 2nd to see the Wallace Memorial, the Hogarth medical paintings ... and the Pathology Museum at the Royal London with the rather well known forensic pathology exhibits and the Elephant Man.' John appeared to be reaching out, building bridges.

On the 29th, I faxed Rod Daniels to ask that Dr Longyear attend our meeting: 'Dr. Longyear ... sits on the Board of Directors of Longyear Corporation. The excavation technique, that Charles will discuss, may involve Longyear Corporation. Things may have come full circle. J.M.

Longyear started the town of Longyearbyen. Eighty years later, we may use a technology of Longyear Corporation.'

At last an answer came to explain Jeffrey Taubenberger's wavering attitude to the project. On a Friday afternoon, Jeff called me about three p.m. He knew that I was leaving for London, just two days later, as he too had been invited to the meeting.

'Kirsty, I hope that you won't think any malice was intended. I thought you should know before it came out in the papers. I thought that you should know before you go to Mill Hill.'

'Jeff, what are you talking about?'

'Last summer, I was approached by Dr. Hultin. You know who Dr. Hultin is, don't you?'

Of course, I knew who he was. He had been Dr Albert McKee's student, from the University of Iowa, who had journeyed to Alaska in 1951 to exhume Spanish flu victims.

Jeff continued, 'Dr. Hultin was impressed by our (Jeffrey and Ann's) work. And he offered to go back to Alaska in order to exhume flu victims. I asked him when he could go, and he said next week. He did go. He brought back samples. We've analyzed them. Remember when I said that I had new cases at the NIH meeting; the cases were from Alaska. I wasn't allowed to share that information at NIH.'

I couldn't respond. Jeff had worked with someone else, behind my back, while being a member of my team. After a moment of silence, all I could say was, 'What permission process did he go through?'

'He went to Teller and asked permission of the elders.'

I thought of my sixteen-month wait for my first permission from the Directorate of Cultural Heritage. I thought of the seven months' wait for the second.

'What safety precautions did he take?' I asked. And this time, I thought of the 4½ years of work that went into planning our project. I thought of the 1½ years that the team had spent in developing safety protocols. Jeff didn't answer my question regarding safety. He told me that he had had Hultin write a letter to him explaining that he (Taubenberger) was not part of the exhumation procedures and was only receiving samples.

Taubenberger volunteered that Hultin had 'little respect' for our project. Hultin thought that my team was wasting time planning and throwing away money. He also thought that our safety protocols were ridiculous.

Jeff said that he had wanted to tell me all this at NIH, but his boss wouldn't let him. I thought of how I had had to justify the project to NIH. I thought of all the questions that Rob was asked regarding safety. Surely, NIH would have something to say about the Alaskan expedition, planned in only one week. Jeff explained that the media embargo would be lifted on 3 February, the day of the team's conference in London – a pure coincidence, he added. Perhaps I would learn more of the secret expedition when the papers covered the story.

I hung up the phone and looked blankly at my parents, who had been privy to my side of the conversation.

'What are you going to do?' my mom gasped.

'Go for a run.'

A run would allow me to think, to contemplate Jeff's actions, and to plan how I would break the news to my team.

9 Mill Hill Meeting

February 1998

Early Monday morning I arrived, two large suitcases in hand, at an old bed and breakfast on a quaint street in London, England. In the parlour sat Les Davis and Alan Hegginbottom, waiting patiently for Charles Smith and Peter Lewin. Les was recounting his previous night at the Oxfords' and how he had perhaps misjudged John, as he had had such a pleasant evening at his home.

'Hi folks!' I said, and I gave each of my friends a hug. 'I hate to interrupt, gentlemen, but I have some rather disturbing news,' I said.

'Is everything okay? Are you okay?'

'I'm fine. It's the project. There've been some developments – as of Friday, actually. I wanted to tell you all in person.' Peter and Charles quietly took a seat.

'What's going on?' Charles asked.

'Friday afternoon I received a call from Jeff,' I began. I then quickly shared all the details of my last phone call with Dr Taubenberger – I no longer thought of him as Jeff. He was Dr Taubenberger. As I revealed each new fact, I watched my colleagues' – my friends' – faces cloud over.

'The sneaky ...,' Alan blurted out. Charles just hung his head and repeated, 'I can't believe it. I can't believe it.' And Peter, always the gentleman, simply said, 'I am surprised that that nice young man would work behind our backs like that.'

'It's a lot to take in ... I'm sorry. I've been planning how to tell you all; but there really is no easy way to break the news ... I am still in shock, and I've known for several days now.'

Alan asked, 'How can he get away with it? It's downright devious.'

'Never mind that. Dr Hultin may have broken the law,' Charles said.
'What do you mean, Charles?' I asked.

'Dr Hultin would have been required to involve the state medical–
legal authorities. Kirsty, did he do that? Also, you said he was a retired
pathologist from San Francisco, right? He had to be a licensed physician in Alaska.'

'Charles,' Alan said, 'maybe in Canada that's the law. Maybe it's different in the United States.'

'Alan, he would have to have been licensed.'

'I don't know if he contacted the legal authorities,' I said. 'Dr
Taubenberger said that Dr Hultin did not contact anyone in Brevig,
Alaska, because he wanted to discuss the exhumations with the villag-
ers in person, as the implication of his work was sensitive. After reaching Brevig, Dr Hultin gained the support of a member of the village
council. The village council was called together in order to decide
whether or not Dr Hultin should proceed and the council agreed that
he should.'

Peter, always sensitive to Aboriginal issues, respected the fact that
Hultin gained the support of the local community. But Charles pointed
out that Hultin was still required to respect the law. Charles was right.

A year and a half after our discussions in the London B&B, I contacted the Alaska medical authorities to find out the state's rules for
exhumation; I needed the information for a talk that I was preparing.

Anyone undertaking an exhumation is required, according to the
state medical examiner, Dr Propst, to respect Alaska's statutes and its
Administrative Code. 'Alaskan natives' and 'non-aboriginals ... have
the same rights, dead or alive. There is no statute discriminating
between the groups.'[1]

Hultin was required to obtain a permit before disinterring any body
(native or non-native), according to the current Alaskan Statutes (AS)
18.50.250.[1] Request for permission should have been made to the state
registrar, according to the Alaska Administrative Code (ACC) 05.540,
or to the local magistrate, who had been delegated authority. The local
registrar for issuance of permits for bodies at Brevig Mission is the
magistrate, Nome Trial Courts. According to the magistrate, 'During
and after 1996, no permits were issued for disinternment [sic] and reinternment [sic] at Brevig Mission.'[2] However, disinterment may also
occur through court order in lieu of a permit, if 'necessary for an official investigation. The events in August, 1997, at Brevig Mission do not

appear to qualify as such an investigation, but on occasion in the past disinternment unconnected with official investigations has been requested through and ordered by the courts under that regulation. Superior and District Court records at Nome do not show any such filings or orders for disinternment or reinternment at Brevig Mission during the period 1996 to the present.'[2] Although usually such an order would be requested from the courts in Nome, such a request could have been filed in another court location. The magistrate, Nome Trial Courts, has 'no way to determine if a disinternment order was issued in another location, but has no indication that it wasn't, either.'[2] Failure to obtain permission for disinternment is a class A misdemeanour, according to AS 12.55.135, which allows for an 'imposition of up to one year in jail.'[3]

Hultin was also required to be licensed in order to perform an autopsy, according to AS 08.64.160.[4] Failure to hold a licence is a class A misdemeanour.[4] Hultin was a retired pathologist from California. His comments during *Pandemic* are worth noting: 'I needed autopsy tools, but of course being retired I didn't have access to that, so I looked around and I found my wife's pruning shears.' Taubenberger had Hultin write a letter explaining that Taubenberger was not associated with the exhumations and was merely receiving samples.[5]

Les, the team's GPR technician, then asked Charles whether the exhumations in Alaska had been risky. 'I mean, you all have gone to so much trouble about safety precautions. Dr Hultin didn't bother. Did he put the village at risk?'

I jumped in. 'Hultin reasoned that there was no risk of live virus in 1997, as there had been no live virus found in 1951.'[5]

Charles picked up the conversation, 'Yeah, but Hultin exhumed "new" bodies in 1997. It was impossible to know if these new bodies contained live virus.'

'Exactly, Charles,' I said. 'Also, Hultin failed to recognize that these new bodies had new locations – locations with different micro-environmental conditions which might have influenced biological preservation. Alan, as you and Les know, temperature and moisture can vary significantly within a small area; these differences might mean different preservation of a body and different preservation of a virus.'

Charles added, 'The new bodies might have differed in body type and, hence, differed in preservation from the bodies exhumed in 1951.' He explained that an obese victim might have been better preserved than a thinner person. Further, different methods of burial might also have affected preservation – for example, air-drying versus immediate interment.

Dr Hultin's work clearly showed different preservation of victims; skeletons were found near a well-preserved woman. Hultin attributed this preservation to the fat content of the body. Regardless, a well-preserved body was found that contained fragments of virus. My later communication with the Alaska health authorities revealed that, despite Hultin's reasoning that there was no risk of live virus, 'Good sense practice would have recommended his consulting with the local epidemiologist and state medical examiner for Alaska prior to disinterment, as bodies of Spanish flu victims are potentially infectious.' There was no consultation.[4]

Our conversation continued. 'Charles,' I said, 'both Dr Hultin and Dr Taubenberger concluded that there was no risk of live virus, yet Dr Taubenberger gave Dr Hultin a preservative which would have killed any living virus. If they truly believed that there was no live virus, why did they need a virus-killing solution? If they argue that it was for safety reasons, why didn't they take any safety precautions during the exhumations?'

Les interrupted, 'You haven't answered my question. Was there a risk to public safety?'

Charles said, 'After concluding that there was no risk of infectious virus, Hultin concluded that there was no risk to public safety.'

Les repeated, 'You're not answering my question, Charles. Was there a risk?'

'Les,' I explained, 'our team found the risk of finding live virus to be extremely low in the Svalbard samples because ground temperatures over the last 80 years, as ascertained by Alan, had been found to range between –4 and –10°C. The infectivity of influenza viruses is not stable for extended periods in the temperature range of –18 to –4° C; and influenza viruses are conventionally stored at –70°C to maintain infectivity. However, the team recognized that the possibility of infectious virus in tissue could not be excluded and was considered a risk of the project. The team also recognized that a potential virus was a level-4 virus and that all laboratory studies would have to be conducted under BSL 4 conditions. The expert panel at the December NIH meeting estimated the risk of finding live virus to be 10^{-18}. Despite the minuscule risk, it was agreed that the risk, a level 4 risk, could not be ignored.'

Charles continued: 'Our team concluded that there was a risk of finding live virus, and hence, there was a potential risk to the public; therefore, safety measures had to be taken.'

A later examination of the published material on the Alaska expedition would reveal the following: one of the village elders asked if Hultin needed help and offered him the services of four young men. Hultin and his assistants began to dig in the open air. The group worked without precautions because Hultin believed that the virus was dead, as it had been 46 years earlier in Brevig Mission. Hultin wore gloves, but that was only to keep his hands clean.

On the afternoon of the third day, Hultin discovered the body of a well-preserved woman. He took tissue from the lungs of three other bodies nearby; however, these bodies were badly decayed. Frozen lung tissues were biopsied from each in situ, and tissues were placed in formalin, alcohol fixatives, and RNAzol (Tel-Test, Friendswood, TX).[6] Five days after the group began the work, they began to close the grave site.

Hultin then took his samples back to San Francisco in an insulated and refrigerated pack. They were then sent to Taubenberger in four separate packages via Federal Express, United Parcel Service, and the United States Post Office's express mail.

My last thought at the London B&B: 'I guess there's no point discussing the Alaskan expedition. It's finished. What matters is how it will impact our expedition. I mean, is there any point continuing our work if Dr Taubenberger is getting answers from Alaska?'

'You're damned right,' said Alan. All heartily agreed that we needed to continue.

'If that's the case, I guess we should make our way over to NIMR. I might as well tell the others the news before tomorrow's meeting.'

At NIMR, in Mill Hill, there were hugs, hand shakes, and hellos all around, and then my news.

'The ... the dirty ...' Rod Daniels exclaimed. 'Taubenberger waited to see if he had results from Alaska before he told you, didn't he? If he didn't have results, he was still part of your team. And if he did have results, he beat you to the punch. The dirty ... Have you told Sir John?'

'No.'

'Come on, I'll take you. He should know; he'll be absolutely steaming. We should issue an immediate press release and beat Jeff to it.'

'That's what the others want, too.'

'Kirsty, here it is.' He opened the door.

'Hello, John, it's nice to finally meet you.'

'You, as well. What seems to be the problem?'

'Well, there's been a little surprise.' I recounted the story for the third time that day. Sir John was unfazed, 'So let him go. We don't need him. We can certainly do it ourselves.'

'The team wants to issue an immediate press release.'

'No, I'm against that. There'll be no statement.' It was not his decision to make. The team operated according to democratic principles, and there was a clear majority in favour of a press release.

'Dr Taubenberger would like to talk to the group tomorrow and explain,' I repeated.

'I'm sure he would. I don't think it is appropriate though. Do you?'

'Well, some information might be useful. We will once again be asked how we can rightly go ahead with our project in light of Dr Taubenberger's new work. We need to know what was done in order to answer properly any questions from both the Norwegian authorities and the press.'

'Well, perhaps Jeff can fax the team the embargoed release.'

On 2 February 1998, Dr Jeffrey Taubenberger faxed me for the last time: 'I would have preferred to talk to the group about our work, but since that is not possible, I am forwarding two press releases that describe the work. The information contained in them is embargoed until Thursday, 5 February, 1998, 2PM EST. We felt it was however important that this information be made available to your group for your discussion tomorrow. The decision to release information about the Alaska case was in the hands of the city council of Brevig Mission, and they gave permission for the press release only last week.'

Taubenberger wanted to talk to our team now – six months after Hultin's exhumations and two months after the NIH meeting (where he spoke against our work). He made it clear that he was finally severing relations with our team; he no longer needed our samples, he had secured permafrost samples of his own. He referred clearly to 'your group,' as opposed to 'our team.'

The embargoed release read in part: 'In August 1997, pathologist Dr. Johan V. Hultin asked the City Council ... for permission to exhume victims of the deadly 1918 "Spanish" influenza. Brevig Mission was devastated by the flu pandemic in November, 1918, losing approximately 85 per cent of its population in a single week. According to church records, the victims were buried in a mass grave at the Mission cemetery.' Hultin had participated in a similar effort. 'The 1951 expedition, carried out by the scientists from the State University of Iowa, sought to culture live virus from victims of the Spanish flu buried in permafrost. No live virus was found and molecular genetic analysis of the samples was not possible at the time. In the 1997 expedition, he hoped to recover lung samples that retained genetic material from the 1918 virus.'

'City council approved the work and lent valuable support to the project in the hope that the tragedy that befell their community eighty years ago could yet contribute to understanding the basis of the disease. Dr. Hultin conducted the exhumation from August 19–24. In the permafrost layer remains of eleven victims were identified, of which four retained soft tissue. The bodies were not removed from the permafrost and lung biopsies were taken directly from the frozen remains. The samples were placed in fixatives that preserve genetic material while destroying live organisms. Dr Hultin contributed the samples to the Armed Forces Institute of Pathology [AFIP] where scientists in the Molecular Pathology Division were already conducting genetic analyses of the 1918 virus from fixed archival tissue samples. Because similar samples in 1951 provided no live virus, it was decided that it was exceedingly unlikely that live virus would be present. Therefore no attempt to culture influenza virus was made.' After the exhumations, 'Dr Hultin oversaw the restoration of the site and built replicas of the two original 1918 wooden crosses. He gave a lecture on his work to the high school students who then helped with placing the new crosses at the grave. A bronze plaque with the names of the 72 victims will be engraved and mounted on a larger cross.'

AFIP itself issued a news release: 'Hultin sent samples from four Brevig Mission victims to the AFIP in guanidinium thiocyanate, a solution that preserves genetic material while inactivating any live organisms. One of the four victims' samples yielded genetic material of the 1918 virus. The AFIP archives were the source of the first case to provide a direct look at the virus, as reported in Science in March 1997. Recently, another positive case has been identified by screening formalin-fixed, paraffin-embedded tissue samples from the AFIP archives. Both archival cases were autopsies of U.S. servicemen who died during the pandemic – the first in Fort Jackson, S.C., the second in Camp Upton, N.Y.'

Taubenberger reported: 'While the RNA, the genetic material of the virus, is fragmented into tiny pieces in all three cases, molecular techniques can be used to identify complete gene structures. All three cases are from the lethal fall wave of the pandemic. Available records indicate that all three victims died within a week of infection. "Analyses of three cases from geographically separated areas will allow us to evaluate the genetic variability of the pandemic virus strain," said Ann Reid, molecular biologist at the institute.'

Taubenberger had his samples. AFIP was getting results. But the state medical examiner of Alaska said, 'I can't believe that this happened in my state without my knowing. Are you sure that there were exhumations?'[4]

On reading the two releases, my team members were adamant about issuing their own media alert. However, the decision was the SAG's to make. Four SAG members wanted the release; Sir John was against it, and Rob Webster was unavailable for comment. Because the majority favoured it, I was responsible for producing a suitable statement.

We Canadians returned to our B&B, and Charles and I sat down at his lap-top computer. After typing out a first attempt, we left, release in hand, for dinner with the rest of the team. Before dining, however, I presented the document to the SAG, which approved it. Sir John, however, was still strongly disapproving.

In response to Taubenberger's releases, the team wrote about the unpublished results of the GPR study of October 1997 and about the exhumation procedures being planned with the strictest safety and ethical standards.

The next morning I was up early. I faxed the release to *Svalbardposten*, Reuters, Canadian Press, and Associated Press as requested by the team.

Later, Hultin commented on our work. On 3 March, Rod Daniels faxed me about an article that he had read on the Alaskan expedition: 'There were a couple of "not nice" comments in that he (Hultin) wanted to remove all obstacles and do things quickly unlike the international Svalbard project which had been three years in the planning, and Kilbourne and Cox were congratulatory on the finding of more 1918 positive samples.'

Drs Edwin Kilbourne and Nancy Cox had been approving of the work. Both flu specialists had served on our expert panel at the NIH, to which Rob Webster had given details of our team's safety protocols and answered questions about our protecting both the environment

and the nearby population. Hultin had admittedly taken no safety precautions. And Kilbourne and Cox were congratulatory.

One Canadian team member summed up the situation – 'We had to
do it right; the Americans just had to get results.'

Meeting, 3 February

Five minutes before the NIMR meeting on 3 February, I spoke privately to Sir John, the chair. 'A number of the team members are upset
because the Necropolis Company is present. I have repeatedly asked
that they not be included in this meeting because they are not team
members. I have previously spoken with John Oxford, Rod Daniels,
and you.'

'This puts me in a very difficult position.'

'I understand that, and I am sorry. But I called and spoke to you
about this last week.'

'Are they really uncomfortable?'

'Yes, they're very upset.'

I returned to the conference room, not sure what Sir John would do.
He entered the room shortly thereafter, welcomed the participants, and
proposed that we agree to the agenda. He asked Necropolis's Dr Susan
Young and Roger Webber to leave the room because they were not
team members, and, after much discussion, it was confirmed that they
should not attend the meeting – a closed scientific gathering for team
members only. It was the third time that John Oxford had invited
Young – once on a conference call, once in Oslo, and now in London –
and that the team had excluded her.

The first order of business: What to do about Taubenberger? The
team unanimously agreed that he could no longer participate in our
project, after he had worked with Hultin – while being a member of
the Spitsbergen expedition. I agreed to write the letter officially severing our professional relationship on behalf of the team. I updated the
team on the correspondence since the GPR study and summarized the
events of the previous four months. I also briefly discussed some
pressing problems – namely, reimbursement of all my administrative
costs, and breaches of the MOU.[7]

I thanked all team members who conformed to the code of conduct
and reminded them, 'The project leader is to negotiate all contracts on
behalf of the team.' I requested that no team members seek contracts.[7]

I next explained, 'Although it is exciting that we have new team members, teammates have to understand that some decisions were taken before they joined the team.' I explained that grant proposals were based on earlier decisions and that we could not change earlier decisions approved by the granting agencies. For example, Smith was responsible for pathology – the protocols were discussed and agreed on at three meetings and formed the basis of the NIH grant application. Moreover, we had discussed the protocols with the Norwegian authorities and the Norwegian public.[7]

'Last,' I said, 'I would like to thank all those who participated in Phase I. I would especially like to thank Mr Heginbottom and Mr Davis for their excellent leadership in the field and their equally excellent report. Although Phase I was a success, I think it is necessary to develop a code of conduct for Phase II, as we had some difficulties, in regard to conduct with the press, and conduct at meetings with government officials.'[7]

Next, Les presented the GPR results, locating the seven graves. Alan then talked about his ideas regarding the planned excavation, exhumation, sampling, and reburial. He covered travel, accommodation, mobilization and demobilization plans, site preparation, excavation drawings, reburial and backfill diagrams, preliminary equipment lists, and site-restoration schedules.[7] He also discussed eight possibilities of what we might encounter:

- seven bodies in seven separate coffins
- seven bodies in a single pit
- a sound coffin with no ice inside
- a sound coffin, but filled with clean, clear ice
- a sound coffin, but filled with ice, and with body encased in ice that is either dirty (containing fine soil particles) or opaque (containing air bubbles) or both
- a damaged coffin, some soil material and ice inside the coffin
- a damaged coffin filled with soil material and ice, with body encased in frozen soil
- no coffins, bodies in shrouds and surrounded by frozen soil.[7]

Each case, Alan explained, would demand somewhat different field procedures. The first case would be the ideal situation but, Alan thought, the least likely. We would need to develop procedures for all eight cases and make the necessary equipment available on site.[7]

John Skehel asked if a specification could be written for the excavation and reburial, which could then be put out for tender. Alan agreed to produce the document.[7]

Charles Smith spoke next. Charles was very interested in a novel approach to excavation – namely, use of cutting technologies. Three technologies might replace or be assisted by the use of jack-hammers – wire saw, plunge saw, and wall saw. 'The advantages of using cutting technologies include speed, precision, ... and excellent restoration. These cutting devices are made by the South African company called Boart Longyear ... The wire saws have been used in permafrost in the Canadian North. ... The Canadian subsidiary of Boart Longyear suggested that their Canadian users might be interested in doing the work for us.'[7]

Despite Charles's enthusiasm, the team was less than receptive. Tom Bergan said that the new tools would mean later excavation – September rather than August – because the ground would need to be harder. Alan said that it would be necessary to insulate the cut blocks from warm air temperatures. John Oxford asked about disadvantages, and Rod answered, 'cost and complications.' The team decided to use jackhammers.[7]

Rod Daniels then suggested that we address the finer points of excavation – for example, where to put the soil. Charles suggested a large, simple structure to keep the exhumations private. He proposed using a tent inside the larger structure.[7]

John Skehel thought that coring would be a mistake. I said that we had permission for coring and must abide by what we had told the authorities. Charles added that full autopsies are extremely difficult and dangerous on a frozen, infectious body. Tom reminded everyone that the cemetery is a protected heritage site and that the team had informed the authorities that it would use coring – there was no point in further discussion.[7]

John Skehel next questioned whether the bodies could be thawed. Charles said that CDC (at the Windsor meeting) strongly advised against that. Sir John added, 'The team could successfully deal with the biosecurity issues but not the human feeling issues.'[7]

John Oxford assessed microbiological safety: 'There exists only a remote chance of recovering influenza virus from tissues of frozen cadavers from 1918. In contrast we anticipate recovering influenza virus RNA from the samples. There may be an opportunity to recover other micro-organisms from the same tissue samples such as ... *Staphylococcus aureus*, and *Haemophilus influenzae*. The Svalbard 1918 samples represent nevertheless a unique resource for an understanding of the pandemic, the role of influenza virus and the role of secondary bacteria.' The team would take core samples 'from the lungs, trachea, spleen, liver, kidneys, and heart from frozen cadavers using a low-speed drill (less than 200 rpm), where aerosols will not be generated. Tissue will remain frozen throughout.' In autopsies at the time, 'Pathological changes (associated with the 1918 pandemic) were noted in the lungs, trachea, and bronchi consistent with an acute viral/bacterial infection, leading to pneumonia and death. Clinically the descriptions of cyanosis and breathing difficulties with serous cough are those symptoms caused by a respiratory pathogen. Although some unusual neurological features of euphoria were noted, there is no reason to deduce that victims suffered from an overwhelming infection of any organ system apart from the respiratory. Optimal sampling [for our project] would be from right and left lung lobes.' Encephalitis lethargica 'could be a rare complication (say 1:1000 incidence). An optimal sample from the 1918 victims would be from the midbrain.'[7]

John Skehel asked if any documentation existed regarding coring techniques and aerosols. Charles said there was not good information, except for that provided by the mining industry. He said that at low rpms, no aerosols are created.[7]

Charles was 'anxious to sample blood; the best chance to sample would be in the heart. The best chance to sample serum would be pleural effusions or in the liver, kidney or spleen.'[7]

John Oxford then asked if we could re-address the issue of autopsy. John Skehel said: 'John, Tom has explained to you that the Norwegian authorities will allow only coring. The issue is dead.'[7]

'Oh, I just thought ...,' said John, before he was interrupted by Sir John, who repeated, 'The issue is dead.'

Rod Daniels spoke next. His notes read: 'Basically, as discussed, there will be at least three sets of samples required initially: (i) to go to Canada (assuming containment IV up and running in time); (ii) to go to USA (Rob Webster to sort out venue in light of Fort Detrick's pulling out); (iii) to go to UK (the facility at Mill Hill should be ready in time as contracts are about to be signed with CRC construction, but failing this we have the backup at the Public Health laboratory at CAMR, Porton Down, which is *non-military*). As a backup, if (i and ii) are not ready in time, all samples can go to (iii) for a dispatch at a later date from the safety of a Containment IV facility.'[7]

Fort Detrick had pulled out? Since we had not heard this information at NIMR, I brought up the issue of the lab, since Rob Webster, who was not present, was to work at Fort Detrick. John Skehel said that it was not necessary to sort out the use of that facility. I wondered, since Fort Detrick had pulled out, if Peter Jahrling had withdrawn.

Rod Daniels agreed to determine what containment facilities and what transportation and permits we would need.[7]

Charles said that the Norwegians would like to be involved in the testing of samples. Peter, always conscious of our hosts, heartily agreed, 'Of course the Norwegians must be involved. How do we get samples to Norway?' Tom agreed to develop plans for transporting samples to Oslo.[7]

Next, the team discussed financing. Noel Roberts, from Roche, explained that Roche contributed £30,000 to Phase I and had earmarked £100,000 for Phase II. John Oxford said, without explanation, that the team would, however, probably receive only £90,000 from Roche, rather than £100,000. Noel continued, 'Roche will require satisfactory protocols regarding safety and ethics.' John Skehel questioned whether Taubenberger's work might affect Roche. Noel said that it would not.[7]

I then discussed my search for funding; I had approached the Medical Research Council (MRC) of Canada and Health Canada for money for the exhumations, but to no avail. Both agencies thought the project extremely interesting, but outside their funding priorities. Health Canada would, however, pay for Canadian testing of any resulting samples.[7]

The media were the last order of business. I explained that the press release had been issued that morning, since four of the six SAG members and nine of the ten team members at the table had wanted the release. An angry John Skehel restated his feelings that the release was a poor idea. I simply said, 'The team's wish was a press release. We have to accept the majority decision.'

Noel Roberts said that Roche could help liaise with the media. Peter Lewin, however, thought that a commercial company would have a different agenda from the team. Charles Smith suggested a professional group within an institution, such as the public relations team at Toronto's Hospital for Sick Children. Noel thought Charles's sugges-

tion a better option than Roche's. John Oxford stressed that our endeavour was an international project centred in Norway. Charles
asked if there was an appropriate PR group in Norway. Tom Bergan
said that he would be very willing to have the Hospital for Sick Children contacted, as it was very well respected and was in my home city;
PR help, Tom suggested, should be in the same city as the PR contact. I
agreed to meet with the hospital's press people when I returned to
Canada.

Everyone agreed that no interviews would be granted and that we
would continue to communicate as a group with the press via press
release. Charles said that 'no interviews' and 'public funding' could
lead to damaging press. He suggested that only Tom and I be available to communicate with the press.[7]

Charles proposed that the team should have a facility in Svalbard,
which could issue a daily release. Tom responded that the governor's
office would have to be kept informed and that he and the PR person
there would work very closely together.[7]

I then asked how we would maintain the sanctity and safety of
the site while still providing open access to all media, including the
documentary makers. Tom suggested access for the Norwegian film
makers, who were to work with British, Canadian, and American
broadcasters, and for National Geographic. This would mean relatively few people in the cemetery, and yet access for several countries.
Tom also stated that we could not prevent others from entering the
cemetery if they sought permission. It was agreed that we should
commit ourselves to the Norwegians and to National Geographic.[7]

I thought that the scientific meeting was over. However, Sir John then
added a new item to the agenda – live virus – perhaps because the
project had received support for live virus at the NIH meeting on 4
December 1997. I explained that attempting to retrieve live virus was
never an aim of this project and that live virus was a risk of the project,
as outlined in the NIH application. However, John Oxford argued that
the aim was to retrieve live virus.[7]

'No, the aim is not to retrieve live virus. I'll remind you, John, that I
started this project. I even had the MOU changed, regarding the issue
of live virus, and I have all the documentation to prove it.'[7]

Tom Bergan, however, expounded that as long as he had been
involved, the objective was to retrieve live virus. Tom said that we
were arguing about semantics. We weren't arguing about semantics,

we were arguing about whether we should try to retrieve live virus. Sir John asked if I could live with Tom's interpretation.[7]

'I told everyone at the NIH meeting (4 December 1997) that live virus had never been the aim of the project.'

Sir John countered, 'It would be negligent not to look for live virus. Can you live with the team's decision?' There was a clear majority: everyone wanted live virus except me.[7]

'I guess that I have some difficult decisions to make.'

'You wouldn't leave the team?' Alan asked.

'I might have to. I told NIH that this project was not looking for live virus.'

John Skehel responded, 'But, Kirsty, we have more information now. NIH is not averse to the team's looking for live virus, as was once thought. We're the virologists; you have to trust us.'

'But I gave my word to all those present at NIH. I won't make my decision immediately; I will take my time.'

John Oxford piped up, 'You should make your decision as soon as possible. You shouldn't leave the team in a lurch.'

'John, I started the project. Do you really think I would put it in jeopardy? I will inform the team of my decision at our next meeting in Toronto.'

'We should take a short break,' said Sir John. 'Dr Christopher Longyear will give a short presentation on his family and Longyearbyen after the break.'[7]

Everyone rushed for the snacks at the end of the long room. I walked sadly to the other end of the room, wondering, 'Is my five-year search for Spanish flu coming to an end?'

'It would be wrong not to look for live virus,' Sir John trailed after me. 'You have to believe us. Listen, if you need to talk, you call me anytime, and we'll discuss the importance of live virus. If we find the virus, we can genetically characterize the virus, the whole virus, in a matter of weeks. If we find only fragments, the work could take years. You've invested too much in this to let it go.'

A few minutes later, Sir John reconvened the meeting, and Longyear provided a lively discussion regarding his ancestor J.M. Longyear.

Following his talk, John Skehel thanked everyone for his or her participation, and we all agreed to meet in Toronto on 15 April 1998.

There was little time to contemplate the team's decision to hunt for live virus, for we were all invited to a party at the Oxfords', where John proudly declared, 'I want to officially launch the project. Please lift your glasses ... To the project.'

'To the project.'

I was alone on the staircase with paintings of Gillian, while John was officially launching the project.

Nevertheless, the team was moving on to Phase II, the exhumations.

10 Is It Safe?

My trip home from London was pleasant, as I spent it eating English chocolate with Les Davis and his son Darren, and we talked little of the project. It was a welcome respite. I would have two months to decide whether I would pull out of the project.

During that period I agonized over the decision, just as I had struggled with whether to proceed after locating the miners' bodies. I polled my family over and over again regarding live virus, and I also questioned my friends repeatedly. Is it ethically right to go after live virus? Were there any guarantees that nothing deadly would be unleashed? And what about my assurance to the NIH meeting that live virus had never been the aim of the project?

In the end, the advice from all those around me was the same: to continue planning for the exhumations and to make my decision just before the workshop in April. With each passing day, I realized I would have more and more information, such as permission from Norway and details on the excavation and exhumation plan, on which to base my final decision.

Second Permission, March 1998

On 9 March 1998, I received written permission for Phase II, exhumations, from the Directorate of Cultural Heritage. Seven months had passed since I had applied. I was very pleased! Once again, I was grateful that the families had said 'yes' to the work and that my case had been handled with meticulous attention to detail. One family had, however, asked that their relative's grave not be opened. I respected and appreciated their decision, as I know the great difficulty that I would have had in making a similar choice.

My second permission read:

> The application for 1998 is a direct continuation of the project in 1997 and the Directorate is of the opinion that there is no need for a similar consideration for this application, as the case has already been sufficiently discussed when the permission was given in 1997. Your application was, however, sent to the Research Council of Norway and to the Norwegian Board of Health for comments.
>
> The Research Council of Norway supports the application, but feels there are some minor questions which they wish to be clarified.
>
> The Norwegian Board of Health supports the application and advises the Directorate to grant permission on the condition that the project analyses the infection risks and is prepared for action if a member of the team becomes exposed to infection. They also want the hospitals in Longyearbyen and Tromso to be notified when the fieldwork will take place.
>
> In addition the Directorate has received a letter from the relatives of ... asking that his grave should not be opened.
>
> ... The Governor feels that this is an important project whose results may have global significance. They feel that there are both ethical and health aspects as well as focus from the media, which require extra consideration.
>
> *The Directorate remarks:*
> 'There should be a detailed plan for the fieldwork and how to take the required samples, so that the Norwegian authorities are sure that due consideration is taken with regard to the cultural heritage and the ethical and health aspects.
>
> 'The Directorate feels that information about the project should be as public as possible.'

The permission continued: 'The work must be carried out with due respect to the deceased and to the environment (churchyard). No bodies shall be removed from the grave, only the necessary samples for analyses. A detailed plan for the procedures during fieldwork shall be submitted to the Governor of Svalbard. The plan shall cover danger of infection, ethics, and consideration to the cultural heritage, and deal with the questions raised by the Research Council and the Board of Health. A strategy for the handling of the Press and TV shall be made and submitted to the Governor for consideration as soon as possible. Pictures of the opened graves shall only be taken as part of the scientific documentation and not be submitted to the press as news pictures.' After completion of work, 'the excavated soil shall be replaced and the surface reconstructed, so that there are no visible traces of the graves having been opened. The project must be prepared to cover expenses if further repair work is needed later.' The team was to send the governor 'a provisional report within 6 months after the end of the season. A final report shall be available at the latest one year after the completion of the work.'

Planning in Earnest

We could immediately begin detailed planning. Tom Bergan was organizing all details in Norway: providing electricity, liaising with two hospitals, and even arranging 'facilities.' One morning he faxed me: 'The Norw. work laws have no special ramifications that will apply to the digging except that a toilet facility must be available. And this can be solved. One of the bigger entrepreneurs has a hut renting NOK 3000 a month. It is movable, can be heated and has a toilet. The toilet could be a water toilet which is what they usually have, but we can put a bucket/chemical toilet in its place and have a fully operable unit. The contents of the bucket would have to be emptied into an incinerable bin.'

Closer to home, Alan Heginbottom was concerned with who would actually excavate. He suggested that our team could find a work crew from Norway, the United Kingdom, or Canada, and supervise the job ourselves; look for local support in Longyearbyen – for example, from the coal company; or let a contract to an excavation or exhumation company to do specified work under our direction. Alan thought the last the best option and prepared a draft request for proposals.

Charles Smith was busy developing exhumation and sampling procedures. John Oxford commented regarding Charles's planned procedures on 24 February: 'Having decided there is virtually no risk of infection from a frozen cadaver we are now free, if we so decide, to lift out the cadavers for more careful sampling on a conventional pathologist table but modified, with, say, a down draught and also collector underneath to trap any "theoretical" microbes etc. The outline as it stands still very much emphasises risk, such as leaving ice on, using rubber dams, etc. This is probably a left over from the Windsor meeting. In contrast I do feel that these precautions are not necessary and importantly could compromise the accuracy of sampling and hence the whole project. ... In fact I was even musing the idea of samples being taken and immediately transported to CAMR (a BSL 4 laboratory in England), where a fragment could be assessed by histology to make sure we have excellent samples. We would know the result within hours and we could meanwhile stabilize the cadavers as regards their frozen state in a fridge.' As for perceived risk, 'Hultin's recent "boy scout" expedition does, if it shows anything, reminds us of his earlier exhumation where absolutely no virus was recovered and therefore at least to himself he felt justified in exhuming without any precautions whatsoever.' The sampling team should include a truly international group of experts. 'You would be crucial but the team could also compose a forensic scientist and a BSL 4 expert.' (Note the paradox: John was insisting that there was no risk of infection, but recommending a BSL 4 expert.) 'In fact the world could be our oyster because this will be an exciting moment.'

John's correspondence dismayed me. First, Charles, a world-respected forensic pathologist, should be only one of a group of experts taking tissue samples. Second, there was, he said, no risk involved in the exhumation. Neither the team nor the NIH's expert panel agreed. Although finding live virus in the bodies was highly improbable, every safety precaution would have to be taken. Third, he proposed, as he had at Mill Hill, removal of the bodies from the grave. Tom had said categorically that this could not take place. I had fully supported Tom, as we had both promised the Norwegian authorities and people that we would not remove the bodies.

On 25 February, John faxed me again: 'The dig and exhumation itself is a minor side affair compared to the sampling. Unfortunately I do feel strongly that we should reanalyse and revisit even at this eleventh hour the question of possible removal of the entire respiratory tract ... In other words our project, in contrast to the Alaska "boy scout" episode and even to J. Taubenberger's formalin fixed samples, could give us much more complete and satisfying data. Finally I am in contact with Roche in Switzerland and there is reason to anticipate phase II of the grant as promised.'

'A minor side affair' indeed. The excavation and exhumations had required two years of preparation, detailed mobilization plans, and rigorous biosafety protocols. John's pressure was wearing. He knew the rules – coring in situ.

I faxed the SAG 27 February: 'I spoke with Professor Oxford this morning ... and I would like to share with you what we discussed. I explained that full autopsies could not be undertaken [by our existing agreements]. We cannot change autopsy protocol, as we have been granted permission and grant money based on core sampling ... The Alaskan bodies experienced freeze and thaw cycles; despite this, it was possible to get viral RNA from the bodies. It is very possible that the Longyearbyen bodies have not experienced freeze and thaw cycles. Therefore, I do not think that we should assume that virus is not present.' It was not possible to alter the sampling team, 'as we have been granted permission and granted money based on Dr. Smith's heading a pathology team ... Dr. Smith is an internationally-renowned pathologist, who leads the only pediatric forensic department in the world. A second member of the sampling team (Mr. Barry Blenkinsop, Office of the Chief Coroner of Ontario, Canada) has done more permafrost exhumations than anyone else in the world.'

On 2 March, John wrote to the entire SAG and to me. 'So at the risk of annoying everyone on the SAG, I would like to carry on ... We need and still have the time over the next 4 weeks to discuss sampling from all angles and be prepared to modify our plans in light of recent events (meaning Dr. Hultin's exhumations). I think our policy of not commenting in public on Dr. Hultin's trip is absolutely correct.'

I thought that my receiving permission from the Norwegians on 9 March, which specified, 'No bodies shall be removed from the grave,' would finally settle the matter of autopsy. Yet on 18 March, John faxed me once more. 'I noted the Norwegian response about sampling and how ambiguous the permission is. My own interpretation is that we cannot remove bodies from Svalbard but we could if we decide on scientific terms to raise them to a tent inside the graveyard.'

I called John. 'John, there can be no more discussion. The issue is dead.' John would look elsewhere. And so Tom wrote to John on 22 March. 'I like your "never take no for an answer" attitude, but when it comes to the Norwegian permission to carry out exhumation, the interpretation is – as I stated before – that we are to take samples from the bodies while they are still in situ. Whatever happens on Norwegian soil it is my medical license and moral standing that is at stake. And I do not want to risk either!' And on 23 March: 'The agreement with the

Norwegian Government means taking samples while the bodies remain in situ and certainly without moving the bodies out of the pit! I trust we will not encounter further rounds of redefinitions about what this means.'

Sure enough, John faxed Tom on the same day that he received Tom's fax. 'If there are very good scientific reasons why we would prefer to remove the cadavers into a tented structure then the SAG should consider this very carefully indeed. Every organization is open to discussion and, I guess, "especially those in a nice small country like Norway." "In situ" could very well mean "within the graveyard."' And he followed up the next day: 'At the risk of annoying you and everyone else I would not like to drop the topic because, as far as I can see we have some "assertions," and "interpretations" about the letter.'

On 30 March John faxed Tom an apology 'out of the blue.' 'I think you are quite right about the Norwegian permission and I have been in error.' At last.

Tom and I weren't the only ones having difficulty with John Oxford. On 25 February, Les Davis, the team's GPR team member, whom we needed to supervise radar soundings during the exhumations, faxed me to say he was upset with the virologists, particularly John Oxford and John Skehel. 'I fully understand, that from a virology point of view, the GPR survey is irrelevant ... 'I think a clear and practical definition of how each of us is going to benefit, both individuals and corporations, who invest in the project, beyond those project members who are virologists, is required.'

Les Davis faxed Tom Bergan 10 March. 'I was ... surprised at the Mill Hill meeting, how Sir John effectively limited our potential to getting a reviewed paper out of the survey results. ... He was definitely against the paper going for formal review because "it might be interpreted differently." I am certain that we will be able to say the same for the virology results! We are all highly experienced professionals in our respective fields and therefore we should respect each other and put some trust in our interpretations based on our experience. ... I hope finding traces of the 1918 virus will be easier!'

On the same day (30 March) that John faxed Tom an apology, I contacted Dr Harvey Artsob of Health Canada for a written commitment that his laboratory would analyse any tissues that might be obtained from Svalbard. That day Artsob confirmed, 'We are still interested in participating in the project with respect to laboratory testing of tissues from exhumed bodies. We will focus on trying to isolate virus but will use molecular biological analytical procedures as well. We also have an interest in testing the tissues for the possible presence of bacterial agents. All testing done in the Winnipeg facilities will be done using our own financial resources.' Rob Webster had confirmed 18 March that USAMRIID would also analyse samples. 'Thank you for nudging me about the site for conducting studies in a BSL 4 facility in the United States. I have a letter of agreement from the BSL 4 facility at Frederick (USAMRIID) that was enclosed with the National Institutes of Health grant request.'

On 1 April, Tom Bergan faxed me his excellent draft of procedures – a planning document of very high calibre. It included wonderful material from Alan regarding excavation, had detailed information from Charles about exhumation and sampling, and involved risk assessments and biological safety information from John Oxford. Two years of thought, planning, and writing by numerous team members formed the basis of Tom's plan.

I was very thrilled – the team was truly on its way! But how long would the SAG take to approve the document?

While meticulous planning continued, I began to tackle the media issue, as required by my Norwegian permission. I met on 26 March with PR people at Toronto's Hospital for Sick Children. I reported to the SAG: 'I have met with both The Hospital for Sick Children (HSC, or, affectionately, Sick Kids) and the University of Toronto (U of T) PR people. Sick Kids has declined to take on the project, since, as they said, (1) they had had only two international stories, and (2) they would find it very difficult to prevent team members from talking to the press.' The second point resonated for me. 'U of T is to present me with a proposal outlining what they can do for the team by the end of next week ... I would like to suggest the following. First, the U of T PR people be invited to our April 15th, 1998 meeting at the end of the day (i.e. after the scientific meeting). Second, National Geographic and the Norwegian Broadcasters (NRK) be invited to present at the end of the day.' Tom and I had been negotiating with National Geographic and NRK (documentary film makers) in good faith on behalf of the team and at the team's request; moreover, the team had decided to commit itself to both organizations at the Mill Hill meeting.

John Oxford faxed me on 30 March: 'I had a meeting with Hill & Knowlton (a PR firm) agency on Friday about flu in general but we discussed our 1918 project. ... They will be writing to the SAG to explain their position.'

Documentary requests poured in almost constantly, just as they had done since May 1996. There wasn't even a hiatus during my negotiations with Associated Producers. By late November 1997, when negotiations had failed with AP, I began communicating on behalf of the team with National Geographic. The International Group – British, Canadian and U.S. public broadcasters – via John Oxford was clearly stepping up the pressure. It had contacted our SAG as a group since I had made it very clear that I (as instructed in November 1997) was negotiating only with National Geographic, and Tom, only with the Norwegian Broadcasters (as agreed at Mill Hill).

I faxed Governor Ann-Kristin Olsen to see if she would be agreeable to the arrangement to which the team had agreed. Tom later informed me that she was pleased.

As a result, on 11 March, I faxed team members the good news that – since they had committed themselves to National Geographic (both the television documentary and the magazine) and the Norwegian Broadcasters – they now also had the support of the governor's office and the Directorate of Cultural Heritage. Tom faxed me on 18 March: 'the group passed the motion at our meeting in London that National Geographic would be our magazine and that National Geographic and NRK would have priority as regards TV. However, we cannot block interested writing or photographing journalists who would like to have bona fide pieces of information.' On the same day, Rob Webster faxed Rod Daniels, 'I have great concern about the media questions and these must be resolved for the health of the project. It is important that National Institutes of Health (NIH) support is dependent on no preference being given to anyone.' NIH wanted complete access for all journalists. But this project was being run in Norway under Norwegian law, and my team would have to respect the wishes of our host country. The Norwegians were pleased with the media plan.

Decision

While correspondence continued regarding public relations and media, I decided that I would have to live with the decision to go after live virus, as I felt it impossible to delay the expedition or to assemble a new team (which would look only for genetic material); the expedition had already been delayed, and the team members had changed several times to date. Another change, and Norway would have rightly questioned our credibility and ability.

I also had to make sure that the promises that I had made in Norway would be kept. I was concerned that some of my team members' comments were not in keeping with my promises. Furthermore, our team operated according to democratic principles. I had to accept the majority decision, as I was the only member of our team to argue against live virus. I would repeatedly remind myself that half the expert panel at the NIH supported live virus. Isolating a live 1918 Spanish influenza virus would allow the scientific community to: determine the pathogenecity of the virus; prepare vaccines accurately, based on the sequence of the haemagglutinin, neuraminidase, and other genes in the event of the recycling of the 1918 strain; and determine whether the virus would be sensitive to the currently available anti-viral drugs for influenza (such as amantadine and rimantadine) or to the neuraminidase inhibitors. (However, finding only fragments of the 1918 virus would require reconstructing nucleotide sequences, and questions would remain as to how accurately the reconstructed sequences reflect the virus from 1918 and how representative they are of the virulent virus.)

Moreover, Sir John Skehel, one of the leading influenza virologists in the world, said that it would be negligent not to try for live virus. Our expedition would be the only attempt at recovering the samples from Svalbard. We had to do everything in our power to recover as much information as possible.

I would tell my team in Toronto that I was staying with the project.

11 Scientific Plan

April–June 1998

Toronto Meeting, April 1998

The team met at the University of Toronto for the day on 15 April 1998. It was our last chance to gather before the exhumations in Longyearbyen in August. We had an incredible amount of material to pore over – first, the easy decisions: personnel, dates for Phase II, and bookings for travel and accommodation.

And then we had the difficult decisions, all requiring considerable discussion: for example, the contract for the excavation itself. Alan Heginbottom had done considerable research regarding funeral and exhumation companies, following the Mill Hill meeting, and recommended the Necropolis Company for the excavation. Should the team ask Necropolis to perform the excavation? If so, Necropolis would have to take direction from Tom Bergan, Alan Heginbottom, and Charles Smith and would have to meet the requirements of the dig (that is, no disturbance outside the cemetery, no wheeled or tracked vehicles, and so on). Pricing would need to be agreed on for mobilization, demobilization, basic work rate, standby rate, equipment, and shipment. And we would also have to discuss and agree on final wording of the contract and an acceptable payment schedule.

Equipment lists would need to be prepared. Who should prepare them? Should Necropolis be responsible for the excavation list under direction from Tom, Alan, and Charles? Should Tom and Charles be responsible for the exhumation and sampling lists? By what date should the required lists be ready? Who should arrange procurement – renting/buying of equipment – and *carnets* (customs permits) for the equipment to Svalbard? Who should arrange return shipments?

We also needed to produce a detailed site plan and excavation plan. Should Alan develop a site plan, showing all the work areas, structures, facilities, site access, and so on? If so, he would need to know about tent structure and flooring materials. By what date should he have the plan ready? By what date should Tom arrange the electric power supply for the cemetery?

There were also numerous questions to answer regarding the exhumations and site workers. What protective clothing and air supply system should be used? What tissue samples should be taken? What size samples (length and diameter)? How many samples from each organ?

The above questions represented only agenda items 1–9. There were an additional nine items. It was an ambitious schedule! With a tight timeline and difficult decisions, the discussions were often heated. However, there was, as always, Peter Lewin to smooth tensions. Peter, wanting to welcome the team members to his city, had arranged for an Ontario artist to produce a beautiful, sleek, soapstone bear for each member.

Despite Peter's kindness, tempers raged. Part of the anger focused on Dr Jeffrey Taubenberger. John Oxford and John Skehel did not like my farewell letter to Dr Taubenberger. John Oxford thought it 'too soft.' They asked for a follow-up, seeking confirmation that Taubenberger was indeed no longer associated with the project.

The team agreed on Necropolis for the excavation and that Alan, Tom and I should travel to London to sign a contract with the company. We also agreed that the team 'take four sets of samples for labs in the United Kingdom (National Institute for Medical Research or CAMR, Britain's existing BSL 4 laboratory), United States (USAMRIID), Canada (Winnipeg), and Norway' and that the 'samples go direct to final destination laboratories, with couriers: for example, Charles Smith for Canada.'

Sir John refused to discuss the laboratory analyses, as he said that they were a technical issue and that the same processes/methods would be used in all labs. The other specialists had all committed themselves from day one to complete sharing of information. Alan had shared detailed knowledge about permafrost, GPR, and excavation techniques, and Charles, great amounts of material regarding autopsy. Sir John, however, clearly did not subscribe to the team's principle. Did he, like the other virologists, believe that 'a geologist could never understand what a virologist does'?

I wasn't about to let the issue die. 'John,' I said, 'from the very begin-

ning, this team has agreed to complete sharing of information. I would
like to know what techniques will be performed.'

'I don't think that the techniques are relevant.'

'I think that they are very relevant. Having an understanding of the
later virological analyses might help Alan, Tom, and Charles plan the
excavation and exhumations better.'

'They will not.'

'Regardless, I would still like to know what tests will be undertaken.'

'We will test for live virus, and then PCR (an analytical testing
method for viral DNA).'

John Skehel was annoyed by my questioning. He offered to draft a
specific sub-agreement to deal with prompt inter-lab communication,
correlation of results, and release of information. I wondered if he
really wanted 'inter-lab communication,' as he clearly did not want
inter-team communication. He explained that all labs receiving samples would have to sign the agreement, including Fort Detrick, Winnipeg, and Norway.

At the end of the scientific meeting, we had invited the University of
Toronto (U of T) public relations representative and a crew from
National Geographic to present what they envisioned in terms of PR
support and documentary and magazine coverage of the project. John
Oxford was outraged, despite his knowing of the invitation since
26 March. He demanded to know why Hill & Knowlton had not
been invited.

I explained, 'Because the team agreed at Mill Hill that they didn't
want Hill & Knowlton. The team wanted the Hospital for Sick Children or the University of Toronto. Sick Kids declined because they did
not feel that they could prevent team members from speaking out of
turn. U of T will be here later.'

'I want Hill & Knowlton,' John Oxford stammered. He then turned
to Sir John and said, 'John, you know what Hill & Knowlton can offer.'

Sir John, agreeing, suggested, 'We should try to get Hill & Knowlton
here for the end of the day.' Such reversals of decision were par for the
course.

'Once again,' I said, 'the team asked for the University of Toronto. I
do not think it is fair to invite another group at the last moment. I am
afraid that I cannot agree to your request.' But the team suggested that

we hear from Hill & Knowlton as well. John Oxford called a local branch of the firm, and asked for a speaker. I wondered how much advance notice it had actually received.

Hill & Knowlton, National Geographic, and the University of Toronto presented their proposals vis-à-vis our production of the requested document for the governor of Svalbard, detailing how we would liaise with the media in Longyearbyen. John Oxford exploded at the National Geographic crew. 'There is no agreement with you. I don't know why you have come. We won't let you into the tent!' I spent dinner at the Faculty Club of the University of Toronto that evening trying to make amends. I cancelled my next day's trip to Myrtle Beach with family to take the crew out to breakfast. Charles kindly offered to take our British guests, including John and Gillian Oxford, to Niagara Falls the next day before their flight home.

Despite John's behaviour, National Geographic later sent thank-you letters to all participants. John wrote to me on 20 April: 'Congratulations on chairing a very productive meeting in Toronto. Against all my expectations you pushed the 18 point agenda forward so fast that we had excess time! It seems that we now have a clear scientific plan and a document to present to National Institutes of Health (NIH) and Roche ... made for an uneasy few minutes with National Geographic. However they must be used to such changes of direction. The proposal of a defined PR group of Hill & Knowlton and University of Toronto will give the international perspective to the work and should satisfy NIH and Roche.' Nothing had, however, been decided regarding any joint venture.

Planning in Detail, April–June 1998

After everyone returned home, planning continued for Phase II. Rod Daniels faxed Alan Heginbottom on 2 April: 'In respect of shipping containers there is no problem in getting things to Tromso but thereafter there is 1 boat per month, Tromso–Longyearbyen, and it is heavily booked ... keen to hear from Tom regarding the possibility of using an empty coal boat out of Tromso.' About tenting: 'They (Necropolis) are concerned at using the military frame tents proposed – how will they cope with the weather conditions (particularly wind) and their security might easily be breached. Whilst not insisting on using the Field Mortuary tent, such tents have been used at disaster sites all over the world under a plethora of conditions. They are very stable in their own right, further lashings are supplied ... In addition the Field Mortuary tents are supplied with temperature control which may be important in terms of cooling as we have moved things forward to August and heat generated inside the tent with use of lighting, power tools and personnel. Having said this it would still be useful to have the military tents as back up.'

Tom was organizing hotel accommodations and making changes for the governor to his thorough excavation and exhumation plan. Tom faxed me on 23 April regarding his document, soon to be submitted to the governor: 'On p.1 of the "Procedures of exhumation" ... I have written you as "Professor," John Oxford has corrected to "Dr." Please inform me as soon as at all possible whether the suggestion that Professor for the two of you (Kirsty and Charles) should be exchanged with Dr. If your position is Assistant, Associate or full Professor, then Professor is appropriate.' In Britain, 'Professor' is usually used only for the head of the department. Neither Charles nor I was a head, so John had 'corrected' our titles to 'Drs.'

Tom faxed me later the same day: 'Two additional tents have been booked. Cabin has been booked ... The Hospital burns disposables and does not release chemicals in waste water, which goes untreated into the sea. Electricity supply is available from line running along the road, but we need to have clarified the position of the cabin before contract re. electricity is signed.'

On 8 June, Tom booked the team's tickets from Oslo to Longyearbyen.

As the Toronto meeting had requested, Alan completed the team's 'Request for Proposals' for the excavation and exhumation, and he faxed it to Necropolis on 27 April. Two days later, it was suggested that a meeting with Necropolis be scheduled for 21 May. On 1 May, Rod Daniels faxed me: 'As I am sure you have been informed, it (meeting) has been scheduled for 21 May, hope this is OK for you.'

On 13 May, John Oxford faxed me: 'The meeting at Necropolis is scheduled for Thursday morning. We have just received your fax about the horrendous airfare. Please ... get a cheapie.' John faxed me again on the 14th: 'Have you arranged a ticket? I have booked you and Alan into the hotel.' A day later, however, I sent a fax to John cancelling my flight and accommodation because of 'my university commitments and requesting a conference call for the meeting.'

I then called John to explain fully why I couldn't travel. I again asked for a conference call for the planned meetings with Necropolis and with Hill & Knowlton. John agreed to set up both conference calls, although he said a call might be difficult at Necropolis because the company resides in an old building. I suggested that he should perhaps change the venue if a conference call was not possible, as I, as project leader, needed to be present. After more discussion, he agreed to the two conference calls. I rose early 21 May, as London time is five hours ahead of Toronto, and the meetings were starting early. I waited beside my office phone, as John was to call on that phone before the meeting started.

Some time after the first meeting had finished in London, John called me. 'Kirsty, you've been looking for me, I hear. What can I do for you?'

'John, I've been sitting waiting by my phone for your call. Why didn't you do what you promised?'

'It was impossible.'

'But, John ...'

'It was impossible,' he interrupted. 'No facilities for a conference call.'

'Perhaps you could have called me to let me know that. Or, as I asked before, perhaps you could have held the meeting elsewhere. Will there be a conference call with Hill & Knowlton?'

'You can speak to them later. I can't talk now. Alan will fill you in when he returns to Canada.' The phone went dead.

On 2 June, Alan faxed me his notes from the meetings in London. He also wrote, 'I will phone you later today, as there are some things we should talk about.' Some things he seemed not to want to put in writing.

Excavation and Exhumation Plan, 26 April 1998

Tom sent on 26 April, after input from the whole team, the dossier explaining the procedures for excavation and exhumation – with special emphasis on biosafety (see below) – to the governor of Svalbard, Norway's Directorate of Cultural Heritage, and Norway's Health Board, as my permission had requested.[1]

The document[1] specified: 'The actual work of excavation and back-fill is to be done with hand tools (spades, pick-axes, wheel-barrows), supplemented with small power tools, such as electric jack hammers.

No heavy equipment is to be used. A designated Contractor will facilitate the research team in achieving its stated objective ... Tarpaulins would cover a temporary wooden or metal floor, to protect the ground surface from damage or alteration due to the amount of work and foot traffic involved in moving and temporary storage of ground material.' The document estimated that 'approximately 700 m^2 of tarpaulins will need to be spread; approximately 600 m^2 of temporary floor (planks, plywood, metal grid) and walk-ways laid or built; and approximately 30 m^3 of unfrozen soil and 30 m^3 of frozen soil will need to be excavated and moved by wheelbarrow to nearby storage areas, and then afterwards replaced in the excavation pit.' A cabin would 'provide toilet facilities and constitute a shelter.' There would be 'a temporary electric service line' and 'a temporary canvas construction ... above the excavation pit.' Also, 'care will be taken not to expose the ground outside the churchyard, e.g. the area between the road and the yard to unnecessary wear or erosion.'

The SAG 'was to ensure that the exhumation is carried out according to the restrictions specified in the exhumation license from the Norwegian Authorities, and that due respect is paid to the heritage aspects and piety of those interred.' Further, 'preparation of the site, so as to avoid damage to the terrain and features of the cemetery and its environs, will be the responsibility of the Contractor, working under the general technical direction of the Scientific Authority (i.e. Alan Heginbottom). Only the very low number of personnel actually engaged in digging and sampling will be allowed inside the tent erected above the pit. This is motivated by concern that exposure to a potential health hazard is minimized, although any viable influenza virus from the Spanish flu is not considered to be present. Additionally, decorum implies concern for the protected heritage site and piety for the cemetery. Consequently, pictures (still and moving) for public viewing shall not be taken inside the tent erected above the excavation site; pictures shall be strictly for purposes of scientific documentation.'

As for ground work, 'The objective (of the excavation) is to efficiently, yet respectfully, in a manner suitable for exhumation, to expose the coffins and/or bodies of the flu victims in a manner suitable for sampling.'

In doing the excavation, '1. The Scientific Authority will take detailed Polaroid photographs of the 1918 gravesite (especially curb stones and markers) and of all areas of the cemetery and environs that will or may be affected by project activities. 2. Remove curb stones, systematically and numbering each stone, to safe storage. 3. Remove turf from gave site to surface soil storage area, and (if necessary) cover with tarpaulins. 4. For main excavation, move soil to main storage area, protect the sides of the pits from thawing and damage by insulation boards and tarpaulins. 5. Erect protective structures, tents, over excavation, in preparation for exhumation and sampling.'

Jackhammers would break up the ground; wheelbarrows would remove soil and rock to storage areas. 'The excavation, itself, is to be carried out in layers of approximately 25 cm in thickness ... until ... (a) a depth of a few centimetres above the coffins/bodies, as estimated from GPR surveys, is reached; (b) the top(s) of one or more coffins is/are encountered; or (c) the first sign of a shroud or a body is exposed.' As well, 'A 24-hour watch will be organized to ascertain safety and protect both the site as such and equipment.'

The main focus of the scientific planning document was biosafety and the plan dealt with the medically responsible officer (MRO) and his responsibilities, exhumations and sampling, decontamination, retrieval, and transportation of samples. The MRO, Professor Tom Bergan, or his named designate, such as Bjorn Berdal, Charles Smith, or Peter Lewin, would supervise operations. The MRO was to supervise the entire work (digging, sampling, backfilling), ensure proper working conditions, document exhumed remains, and fulfil any conditions in the enabling licence. The MRO was to assure that all staff have the latest influenza vaccine recommended by the WHO and fully understand the nature of the work and potential risks.

The MRO was in advance to assess safety, based on current international strategy regarding infective agents. He was also to inform Longyearbyen Hospital of the project and consult with it on both surgical and medical emergency procedures; the hospital's suite for epidemic disease had an air lock. Tromso Regional Hospital was prepared to assist in any urgent diagnostic work.

Health and safety considerations were paramount for staff involved in the preparation of the site, excavation and exhumations. All excavation and exhumation staff required tetanus immunization, and all staff were warned about possible musculoskeletal injuries and minor skin breaks. Every accident or illness requiring time off work was to be documented and reported to the MRO. Incidents were also to be recorded in the log book, which included a daily time log of all persons entering and leaving the exhumation site.

In the exhumations and sampling, those in close contact with cadavers were to receive prophylactic anti-influenza drugs (Rimantadine) starting the day before first viral exposure and continuing seven days after the last possible exposure. A new neuraminidase inhibitor, with both preventive and therapeutic efficacy in laboratory tests and small clinical studies, was also to be used. During sampling, only the minimum number of people required were to be inside the tent. The autopsy team was to consist of Charles Smith and two assistants. Charles and his first assistant, Barry Blenkinsop, were to carefully open the coffins and obtain samples and were to be considered contaminated. A second assistant, Rod Daniels, was to act as a circulating nurse and was to be regarded as clean. He was to transfer samples into appropriate transport containers. Members of the autopsy team were to wear a Tyvek suit, a water-impermeable barrier, rubber boots, hand protection (latex or Kevlar gloves), and a mask and air-supply system. The coffin lids were to be carefully removed if the bodies had been placed in coffins; the cloth was to be opened if the bodies had simply been wrapped in cloth. There was to be no attempt to remove the bodies from the pits to examine them. Samples were to be taken from only those bodies for which permission had been granted. Tom wrote, 'While dry skeletal remains – naturally aligned or disarticulated – are found in most cases, there may be dry preservation of skin (mummification), or rarely, very considerable preservation of soft tissues even in surprising situations. In wet soil conditions the coffin wood may be well preserved with sodden human remains. From time to time up to one-third of the coffin will contain liquid of decomposition (coffin liquor). The permafrost conditions are consistent with the possibility that water may have filled coffins entirely and that mummification has not taken place.'

A protective barrier (for example, a thick rubber sheet) with small openings was to be placed over the bodies, with the openings over the autopsy sites in a manner similar to the placement of surgical drapes.

Sampling procedures were designed to avoid generating aerosols. Samples were to be taken by means of a hollow coring device. The samples were to be taken through the covering layer of ice. Core samples were to be taken from the lungs, trachea, spleen, liver, kidneys, and heart by a low-speed drill (less than 200 rpm) to avoid formation of aerosols. Tissues were to remain frozen throughout the sampling; however, minimal melting caused by shearing might occur around the bore surface.

In the matter of decontamination, after removal of tissue samples, standard, commercially available solutions would decontaminate equipment and clothing. Disposable equipment and clothing were to be incinerated when possible. All other potentially hazardous materials (such as sharps) were to be disposed of using appropriate containers, consistent with the practices of the medical community in Svalbard.

Reburial followed. Once the samples were taken, the bodies were to be reburied in a safe and respectful manner. Every precaution was to be taken to prevent frost heave of the bodies and to maintain the permafrost. Independent geologists and permafrost specialists were consulted in order to ascertain the best method of burial to prevent resurfacing of the bodies. The coffins were to be covered with 15 cm of fine soil, prepared from the excavated soil, to provide a layer of padding. Excavated soil was then to be replaced in layers 15–20 cm thick, dampened and tamped into place. The pit was to be filled to the original grade level, equivalent to the level of the paths surrounding the grave site. Reburial and backfill procedures had the approval of the local authorities. Monies were set aside should restoration be required later.

Tom's planning document read: 'The objective is to re-store the grave-site cemetery and its environs as closely as possible to their original condition. The Contractor will be responsible for all site clean-up following completion of the work.' Specifically, the contractor would '1. Replace curb stones around the grave site in order, by using maps and the Polaroid photographs, for guidance. 2. Replace fine soil and surface vegetation, so as to reconstruct the gravesite. 3. Re-install grave markers. 4. Re-erect cemetery fence. 5. Remove site protection (plywood, duckboards, tarpaulins, etc.). 6. Fill any post-holes, etcetera, with fine soil. 7. Remove snow fencing from around exclusion area. 8. Clean up all litter. 9. Remove surplus material to approved waste disposal sites. 10. Vacate site.'

Transportation of the samples required that the core samples remain frozen at –70°C; therefore, samples were to be placed in containers providing multi-layer mechanical protection and thermo-protective packaging/encapsulation. The sample material was to be transported by air to a BSL 4 laboratory. After performing tests to establish that there was no viable virus, further tests would be carried out to determine influenza RNA and the presence of bacteria.

It was an impressive planning document. The excerpts presented here give only a snippet of the science and safety protocols. On 12 June, Tom faxed the team that the authorities 'have been rather favourably impressed, apparently, with Kirsty's efforts to present written material and they feel that the additional dossiers they have received this spring are exhaustive.' It was wonderful news. I faxed the team: 'Tom informs me that the Governor is very pleased with the detailed plans. I would like to thank everyone who contributed to the development of the plans. I would especially like to thank Tom for writing an excellent, excellent document. A heartfelt thanks, Tom!'

Now the team just had to write an acceptable PR document, sort out the documentary interests, and pay for the expedition. And then, at last, we would all be off to Svalbard!

12 High Stakes

April–August 1998

Waiting for Sir John

Three months to Phase II, and only a few items stood in the way: namely, Sir John Skehel's promised laboratory agreement – the last piece of the scientific planning puzzle – an acceptable PR plan, and money.

After Sir John offered at the Toronto meeting to write a laboratory agreement, I faxed him (and the remaining members of the team) a reminder of their assigned tasks on 17 April 1998, and soon received detailed submissions. Despite the request, I received nothing from Sir John.

Almost a month later, Rob Webster faxed Sir John: 'You were going to send me a letter indicating that the analysis of samples between the different centres would be a collaboration effort with no pre-publications of any kind – Could you please send me the draft of that letter?' May and June passed, and I received no agreement. Despite Sir John's promise at Mill Hill to be available to answer any of my questions, he was not responding to my requests.

I wrote to Sir John on 13 July, 'A quick note. Has there been any progress on the agreement among labs? I very much look forward to hearing from you as soon as possible.' There was no response. I again faxed Sir John on the 28th: 'I am sorry to bother you with the following request again. However, I very much need an answer. Has there been any progress on the lab agreement which you kindly offered to draft? Please let me know either way.' On 29 July, I faxed Sir John after calling his office. 'I know that you have been away from the office and will not return to the office until later this week. I have sent you several faxes regarding the lab agreement. I know that you are extremely busy. Therefore, I would be delighted to have my own lawyers draft the lab agreement if this would be of help to you.'

Sir John finally responded on 31 July. 'As you can imagine the laboratory agreement is a little more difficult than it might first have seemed. I have discussed it with Rob Webster and although we agree that the scientists responsible for the work described in any paper should take priority, it's more difficult to decide who to include in total because, as yet, we don't even know who will be doing the lab work in Canada. I don't think we should necessarily be in a hurry to do this, so long as it's clear that no publication is made without the agreement of the SAG.'

Why was Sir John discussing authorship with Rob only? Authorship would be a team decision. Equally important, why was he discussing laboratory relations with only Rob? I was pleased, however, to see that he agreed that there would be no publication without the agreement of the SAG.

I knew that the team desperately needed the promised lab agreement, despite Sir John's assertion that we shouldn't 'necessarily be in a hurry.' Very few team members were aware of the broken promises and deceptions, as I had tried to keep team politics as private as possible in order to maintain friendly relations.

I could not imagine the difficulties that might accrue in analysis. The virologists had built their careers studying flu; some had spent their career searching for the cause of the 1918 flu. Careers were at stake, and our expedition was perhaps their last chance for answers. Very few samples of lung tissue existed from 1918, and none might be positive (only one of twenty-eight formalin-treated paraffin block lung samples from persons with respiratory infection from 1918 yielded nucleotide sequences representative of influenza viruses). Moreover, tissue samples had been exposed to formaldehyde, which is known to alter genetic material; and the samples had been stored at room temperature and might be modified. Frozen tissue might provide unmodified sequences of all influenza segments and even – extremely unlikely – infectious virus.

World health was also at stake. It is not known when the next influenza pandemic will occur, but its likelihood increases over time, and it could be as virulent as the 1918 influenza. Establishing the complete nucleotide sequence of the 1918 virus would enable scientists to prepare vaccines in the event of recycling of the 1918 strain and determine whether the virus would be sensitive to anti-viral drugs for influenza or to the neuraminidase inhibitors.

Furthermore, identifying the genetic basis for the high virulence of the Spanish flu would improve global preparedness. If the scientific community understood the molecular basis of high virulence, scientists could identify potential pathogenic strains of viruses very early, before they became lethal on a large scale. Moreover, money was at stake. Flu is big business. Each year, the annual economic cost associated with influenza epidemics is $10 billion in the Northern Hemisphere alone. Annually, influenza infection results in 20–25 million visits to U.S. physicians; and each year, influenza accounts for millions of days lost from work in the United States. And finally, only BSL 4 laboratories, the world's highest-security labs, were to be used to analyse any samples retrieved from Svalbard. Canada's BSL 4 facility had yet to open. Norway did not have one, and USAMRIID, according to Rod Daniels, had pulled out of the project. Any Svalbard samples would have to go to Britain's BSL 4 lab. Once the samples were deemed safe – that is, they contained no live virus – they could be shipped to other labs for further analysis. However, without a lab agreement, I knew that I could not get the precious samples out of Britain.

Therefore, although Sir John had initially offered to write an agreement regarding standardized laboratory procedures, I knew that the team needed a document that would also outline a code of conduct regarding ownership, biosafety, and confidentiality, to which all team members and participating labs could agree.

Toronto Draft, 10 August 1998

On 6 August, I approached, at my own expense, a Toronto law firm about writing a confidentiality lab agreement. The firm produced a draft agreement on 10 August.

> **AND WHEREAS** the Interinstitutional Agreement [our Memorandum of Understanding] sets out that Duncan, in her capacity as a member of the SAG has the authority to enter into contracts with outside parties on behalf of the Institutions involved in the research program;
>
> ...
>
> 1. Laboratory agrees to hold the Property (all samples and any other physical properties in the Laboratory's possession or control as a result of the Research Program), subject to the following terms and conditions:

(a) The Laboratory will keep all of the Property at its laboratories and will not deliver the Property, or any portion thereof, to anyone without the prior written consent of Duncan.

(b) Unless and until the Laboratory has received prior written notice from Duncan to the contrary, the Laboratory will not permit:

(i) anyone other than the authorized employees of the Laboratory to have access to the Property for the purpose of inspecting, analyzing or performing any work therein which has not been authorized by Duncan.

(ii) anyone other than the Laboratory Employees to have access to any of the reports or other materials based on examinations or analysis of the Property;

...

D. The Laboratory acknowledges that in completing its tasks, it will be put in a position of trust and confidence by having possession and knowledge of certain Confidential Information (any information pertaining to the samples, the testing of the samples and the results of the testing of the samples. Any other materials or information related to the samples or activities of the Scientific Company which are not publicly known.)

E. As a material inducement to Duncan to engage or to continue to engage the Laboratory, the Laboratory agrees that the Laboratory shall not, except with the prior written consent of Duncan, at any time during or following the term of the Laboratory's engagement by Duncan, directly or indirectly disclose, divulge, reveal, report, publish, transfer or use for any purpose any of the Confidential Information which has been obtained or disclosed to Duncan as a result of the Laboratory's agreement.

It was an excellent agreement, which recognized my role as project leader, my right to enter into contracts on behalf of the other institutions, and our team's Interinstitutional Agreement.

Since biosafety was the team's top concern, only authorized persons would have access to the property and could not remove it without written consent. I had to make certain that only people with level-IV training would have access to the samples and that the samples could not be removed to another lab (for example, a lab interested in examining the links between Spanish flu and encephalitis lethargica) without my approval. More important, the lab had to agree to take all the necessary steps to maintain biosafety.

I was especially pleased about the provision for confidential information. The agreement prevented labs from divulging any information regarding the testing of samples and the results. This would protect all team members.

Finally, the agreement would be governed by the laws of Ontario. I wouldn't have to worry about Tennessee law.

SAG Responds, 10–13 August 1998

On 10 August, I faxed the agreement to all members of the SAG, and to Dr Harvey Artsob and Professor Bjorn Berdal. I wrote to Artsob: 'I apologize for the impossibly late notice. However, the lab agreement was to be drafted in April; I learned 1 1/2 weeks ago that the agreement had not been written. I therefore took it upon myself, as project leader, to have the agreement written. A Toronto law firm was provided with the Team's Interinstitutional Agreement (IA) and, therefore, the lab agreement conforms to the IA. Please note that this agreement must be signed prior to the samples leaving Svalbard (ideally, prior to my departure on August 14th, 1998).'

Tom, understanding team politics and the urgent need for the document, signed the agreement for Norway's Defence Microbiological Laboratory, as Berdal was away.

On 12 August, Rob Webster faxed me: 'Thank you for pointing out the need for a lab agreement ... We have used your faxed agreement as a model to develop an agreement to be sent to the BSL 4 laboratories. We will send you a copy in the near future. Since this is an important document it will be necessary for the SAG to give their input.'

I responded to Rob on the same day. 'I think that I should provide you with the chronology of events, which led to my contacting one of Canada's top law firms and requesting their services to draft a laboratory confidentiality agreement ... The law firm informed me that such a document is not difficult, but a standard contract. To date, I have had two, direct correspondences – yours and another's (a positive response) – regarding the agreement. Because I have heard indirectly that there is some concern over the document, I would ask that we follow the standard protocols (outlined in the Interinstitutional Agreement) to resolve any difficulties. Therefore, a SAG vote will be taken to either accept or reject the Laboratory Confidentiality Agreement.'

Rob responded the next day: 'Your fax raises major concerns. I do not accept the August 10, 1998 agreement ... We are working on an agreement based on what was sent, and we will send you a copy as soon as the BSL 4 laboratory has reviewed and approved.'

I later asked which BSL 4 laboratory was doing the reviewing and approving; however, I received no answer. And needless to say, there was no future lab agreement from Webster.

After hearing from Rob, I received a three-minute tirade on my answering machine from Sir John Skehel. He disapproved of my sharing with the SAG my numerous requests for a lab agreement from him and my obtaining a lab agreement when his was not forthcoming.

Both Rob and Sir John asked that we leave the agreement until Longyearbyen. Sir John would not sign the agreement for the BSL 4 English lab, and Rob Webster would not sign for the U.S. lab. Tom Bergan had signed for Norway, but the country lacked a BSL 4 laboratory. Therefore the samples could not go to Norway for decoding the virus.

Sign, Canada, Sign

I needed Canada to sign the agreement so that the samples would come here. I phoned Health Canada. I knew that Harvey Artsob would keep his promises to return samples to Norway after testing for live virus and share samples with Britain and the United States. He wanted the samples, but Health Canada no longer did; no reason was given for the change in direction. I called Charles Smith to tell him, and he suggested that I call Peter Lewin, previously a military medical doctor, with 'a friend in a high place at Canada's federal health agency.'

As always, Peter was encouraging. 'Not to worry. I'll make a call. You'll hear from me or someone else very soon, I'm sure.'

I waited anxiously by the phone. A half-hour passed. And then the call. Health Canada wanted the samples again. Peter had negotiated successfully!

But how to get the samples to Canada? Charles had been trying for days to get import permits from Health Canada and Agriculture Canada. Canada's BSL 4 lab was not operational. Without it, there could be no shipping of samples potentially containing a level-4 virus.

Artsob suggested, after speaking with Peter Jahrling, that USAMRIID hold the samples for Canada until the BSL 4 facility was operational. USAMRIID had pulled out of the project but was willing to hold samples for Canada.

I could accept the samples' being held at USAMRIID. If the samples were shipped to the United States and eventually to Canada, I would not need them to be transported to Britain. I guessed that if the team agreed to send the samples to Sir John's laboratory, it would be difficult to return the samples to Norway and to send them to Canada and to the United States (if the labs were interested).

I needed a signature on the law firm's lab agreement. Artsob received permission to sign. Unfortunately, all legal documents had to be reviewed by his legal department. It would take days to get the necessary signature. I was leaving for Longyearbyen in one day.

I could wait for the signature – even in Longyearbyen. However, within the SAG, Sir John and Rob Webster were against the law firm's agreement. Tom Bergan, Alan Heginbottom, and I were for it. I needed John Oxford's signature. Unfortunately, he sided with Sir John.

It was over! The samples would, I knew, go to Britain. I also knew that without a lab agreement, I would have an impossible fight to get the precious samples out of Britain for further analysis.

13 Public Relations Plan

May–July 1998

Public relations continued to be an issue, even after the Toronto meeting when John Oxford had suggested using both Hill & Knowlton (H&K) and the University of Toronto for the project. Roche had offered to pay H&K, London, for the PR campaign, which was to cost £20,000, £30,000, even £40,000, according to Oxford. John had earlier promised me that the money would go to H&K, Toronto, and that PR would be run from my city.

Hill & Knowlton or Not?

H&K, London, faxed me its media-relations proposal on 20 May. On the 28th, John Oxford wrote: 'The vital point is that both our funders NIH and Roche have given us a clear message to take on a professional PR group. There are, fortunately, no funding implications because Roche (quite generously) will foot the extra bill. So as with a very multidisciplinary project, the work is now divided up, [Tom] will take the questions of bacteria, John, Rob and I will deal with influenza per se, Alan with permafrost, Charles with sampling and Kirsty with ethics and the like. ... Thus a single spokesperson is now redundant.'

John was insisting that the project's funders wanted a professional PR group. He was also overruling our SAG decision of September 1997, which designated Tom and me spokespersons for the project.

John continued to urge the team to use H&K, and on 8 June I faxed him in the light of his nudging. 'I appreciate that the SAG is very much in favour of Hill & Knowlton. Unfortunately, it is impossible to make a final commitment to H&K, as (1) the University of Toronto has yet to commit to H&K's proposal.'

On 9 June, H&K faxed me. 'Please contact H&K urgently. I would be very grateful if you could call me or fax me to give me your thoughts/ approval of our proposal. We will also need your decision on the appropriate SAG spokesperson for general contact during the media management programme. Professor Oxford informs me that he and other members of the SAG have been in touch with you to express their approval and that you will be writing on behalf of the whole SAG.'

I responded strongly to H&K's fax on 9 June: 'The University of Toronto is unable to commit to the proposal, as it requires clarification on a number of issues, primarily funding ... I had asked that H&K contact the University of Toronto over a month ago. I am surprised that H&K would put forth a proposal without contacting a major party to the proposal. As I have already explained, I will be the SAG spokesperson for general contact during the media management programme.'

Tom faxed me on the 11th, after speaking with Torsten Hoof, Oxford's contact at Roche: 'After the information from Hoof yesterday and the fax this morning, it would seem difficult for you to find any option but to respond positively to H&K ... I know who calls the shots. You have to accept H&K with your hands tied. (John Oxford is threatening that without H&K, no Roche or NIH funding.)'

I refused to cave in, as I had yet to hear from the University of Toronto, but pressure continued. Sir John's assistant, Marilyn Brennan, wrote on 12 June: 'John Skehel asked me to call you to find out what the situation is as regards to the arrangements with H&K.'

I wrote to Sian Wright of H&K on the 12th: 'The University of Toronto faxed me a copy of the letter to you detailing what they are prepared to offer ... I will contact you Monday morning at 9:00 a.m. in order to discuss the proposal.' On 16 June, Lucy Turvill of H&K wrote to four members of the six-member SAG team. She promised a first draft of the press pack by early July, although I had yet to formally commit us to H&K. On the 16th, I faxed Sian Wright: 'As you know, the SAG is pleased with your proposal. I am delighted to hear that you will be able to work with the University. I would now like to commit to the proposal. However, I require the following commitments from H&K. (1) I am the contact person for the SAG. (2) All communication with the team should be addressed to me only and no one else. (3) ... H&K Toronto should look after the PR for the project.' I wrote to the SAG on the same day. 'The second Roche grant is dependent on our commitment to H&K. (I learned this only last week. This stipulation was never announced.)'

On 17 June, I faxed Sian, thanking her for agreeing to my requirements. However, the London office seemed reluctant to involve the Toronto office. The reason was not obvious until roughly two months later.

John Oxford faxed me on the 17th: 'I am sorry to say that you have misinterpreted my letter and also the spirit of the agreement with Roche. Roche has always maintained a "hands off" position as regards the grant. Roche has always advised the SAG to take professional advice on PR and suggested H&K.' John had previously warned us that without H&K there would be no Roche or NIH funding for the exhumations. Now he was saying that Roche was merely suggesting H&K. But Tom Bergan's June conversation with Torsten Hoof of Roche made it clear that I would have to 'respond positively to H&K.' John Skehel's office also faxed me: 'We have been unable to contact you for the last few days and have prepared the enclosed letter to H&K (London Office) which will be sent to them at 4:00 this afternoon. The Group (i.e. the SAG) is in agreement with the proposals.'

I had received no messages at any of my four phone and fax numbers, or even at my e-mail address. Regardless, John Skehel was going to commit us to H&K if I didn't. I wondered why the director of the NIMR would resort to such tactics. I had after all planned to commit us to H&K, as it had finally spoken with the University of Toronto, had provided me with the commitments that I needed, and had the majority vote of the SAG.

On the 17th, I faxed the team. 'I would like you to know that I committed, in writing, to H&K this morning, June 17th, 1998. H&K in conjunction with the University of Toronto will be looking after the PR for the project.'

Press Pack

The team's next task was to come to an agreement regarding the 'press pack' – a media kit containing information on the project, the 1918 influenza, the team, and the science of the virus.

On 30 June, I received a fax from H&K. 'Work has begun on the press pack so could you ask all SAG members (except Professor Oxford who supplied his biography a little while ago) for their biographies and portrait photos please.'

I received press mock-ups on 16 July 1998. H&K explained that it used 'the historical photos supplied and flu virus diagram to give a montaged image.' The collage of a spiky virus, hospital wards, and death statistics was appalling.

I immediately wrote to another H&K representative, Rachel Allen: 'The following changes must be made to the media kit: (1) The emphasis should be the project ... H&K was provided with a background of the project. (2) The project is not merely a virology project ... The multidisciplinary nature of the project needs to be brought forth. (3) A section regarding respect and dignity for the deceased, the Church and the community of Longyearbyen and the people of Svalbard must be included ... I would be most happy to provide you with this section. (4) The project takes place in Svalbard, Norway ... Information regarding this unique area of the world must also be given. Again, H&K was provided with this information.' On the 20th, I faxed Rachel: 'I sent, via courier, three pictures: (1) the seven markers in the cemetery and two photos of the Church. These pictures ... will provide an ideal cover for the press pack, as the pictures focus on Norway. The current mock-ups are unacceptable. We simply cannot have pictures of the virus and the word "death" on the front of the press pack.'

A message from John Oxford prompted a response from me on 27 July: 'What do you mean that "some interviews are being taken" already? I will remind you that the Interinstitutional Agreement specifically provides that the participation of a member of the project may be terminated for unauthorized disclosure to the media (see section 6 (b)).' John was not abiding by the team's rules, and there was nothing anyone could do about it. My choices were to sue him or to drop him from the team. John knew that I had no money to take him to court – Tennessee court – and team members were very worried about a backlash.

On 28 July, H&K faxed me a new version of the text. I suggested changes. A new version of the text and mock-ups was faxed to me the next day. I responded on the same day: 'I am delighted with design 2 (of mock-ups). Please fax 2 to the other SAG members. We still unfortunately need changes to the document. The cleaner the document, the greater the chance of the SAG's approving it.'

However, while I waited for a corrected version of the press pack, H&K faxed Sir John a copy of the text. I responded to Sian Wright on

29 July: 'I am writing to you in order to express my dismay regarding two breaches of the understanding between H&K and myself ... (1) Sir John should not have corrected the document, as I am your sole contact ... The text does not recognize all team members' efforts. Please be advised that the project is a team effort and that everyone must receive his proper recognition. (2) Sir John Skehel's document should not have been faxed to the SAG members, as I am to communicate with the SAG on your behalf. Furthermore, you were left a telephone message yesterday, July 30th, 1998, indicating that I would fax the SAG when the final, corrected document had been sent to me. I require that the changes be made to the July 30th, 1998 document.'

Tom was equally exasperated with H&K and copied me on his fax to his friend Professor Bjorn Berdal on 30 July: 'Enclosed pls. find last night's "harvest" from the fax regarding the Svalbard project. Sorry that you might miss new faxes from our project pen pals in Turner Street, but I promise that this will be corrected in the near future, so do not despair. Please note that a forward thinking public relations company called H&K appears to have, as one of their highest wishes, a desire to get their hands on a copy of Professor Berdal's CV. They even want a picture – I have sent my CV, but had to decline a picture, so maybe you can send two pictures of yourself – so that they get their quota of Norwegians filled.'

John Skehel faxed Sian Wright on the 31st: 'After our conversation this afternoon about the urgency of getting an acceptable draft to the University of Toronto, you should go ahead with the corrected version that you now have had from me and I'll contact Kirsty Duncan to indicate that you are acting on my authority as representative of the SAG.'

On 31 July, H&K faxed me: 'Please find attached the text for the press pack as amended on the instruction of Sir John Skehel, for your information.' On the same day, Skehel faxed me: 'I have contacted Sian Wright at H&K about the draft of the website and made some alterations to it, together with John Oxford. Since Sian indicated to me that for the University of Toronto this is a real emergency I've authorized her, on behalf of the SAG, to go ahead and submit the modified version to Toronto. I hope you find the modifications acceptable; Sian will now fax them to you and perhaps you could send the correct version to the SAG for information.'

I called Sir John and angrily explained that he had broken our agreement. Surprisingly, on 3 August he backed down: 'I corrected the text because I learnt of its existence from H&K at a time when I knew that I would not be available for the next several days. This was unavoidable and so I thought I could have useful input at that stage.'

Sian Wright faxed the SAG. 'We have now produced a text that has almost been approved by Kirsty Duncan and also, on Friday last week, a text which Sir John Skehel and Professor Oxford are agreed upon. Unfortunately, these two texts are very different.'

On 3 August, Tom faxed Sian Wright: 'Enclosed pls. find numerous suggestions improving the manuscript re. the Spanish Flu project. There are both factual errors and sloppy mistakes in English. Giving us, in effect, only a few hours to correct the manuscript is rather surprising, given the several months HK has been involved and its knowledge that the project D-day is August 16, 1998.'

John Oxford replied the same day: 'As regards to the H&K document I am afraid Kirsty insisted that the SAG should *not* see it until she had provided a version. H&K had a good version weeks ago but Kirsty wanted to add a lot of detail about Svalbard etc. etc. The original document was mainly about flu ... So please do not blame H&K!'

H&K sent Tom's amendments to Sir John. It appeared that H&K required John Skehel's approval for any changes. Sir John wrote to Tom: 'I just received a copy of the text for the website – it's fine. The only things I would question are right at the beginning where you talk about genetic material. We are in fact trying to get the virus.' Tom responded succinctly: 'When we met in London on Feb. 3, we agreed to put our primary goal as genetic material, but that all efforts would be made to isolate the virus. This slight difference of emphasis has been repeated to the Governor, Riksantikvaren and the press!' There was no more discussion.

I tried unsuccessfully to find out who was in charge of Sian's branch but was able, soon after, through the Toronto office of H&K, only to learn the name of Dr Martin Godfrey in London. I faxed him on 3 August to thank him for including the text on respect and dignity, the team's biographies, and the 'Norwegian' cover for the press package.

The section on respect read: 'This project is not just about cold, hard science. It is about seven young men who died tragically like 20–40 million others in the world's worst pandemic. The scientists in the research team have pledged to take time and care to remember these young men and their families ... We recognize that what we asked is potentially very hurtful, as we are largely outsiders asking to undertake something very personal. We are grateful to the families of the young men, the Church of Longyearbyen and the people of Svalbard and Norway.'

On 4 August, H&K sent me a new version of the press package.

H&K's Final Press Pack

On 5 August, Sian Wright wrote to the SAG: 'Attached are the final versions of the 1918 backgrounders. These are the result of over three weeks of discussion between ourselves and Kirsty Duncan, latterly with Professor Oxford and Sir John Skehel and finally with other members of the SAG team. Kirsty has informed us categorically that she has the final say in the wording of these documents and that she has an agreement with the rest of the SAG to that effect. This ends (on Kirsty's instructions) H&K's involvement on the development of the press pack – we have no time, nor do we have any budget to work further on it.' However, H&K had chosen on its own to withdraw.

There would, I believed, be no more correspondence from the company, as it had finalized the document. Tom, angered by H&K's voluntary withdrawal from the project and refusal to correct the manuscript, faxed Sian Wright on 5 August: 'I am shocked that you sent a fax yesterday afternoon expecting everyone to drop whatever obligations they have and devote the rest of the day as per your dead-line a few hours later. I am further shocked to read your divorce declaration/disclaimer covering your fax this noon ... If you have sent this with the uncorrected information about the team as this would suggest, the least you can do is quickly correct the manuscript.'

John Skehel was angry that the press pack would include the section on respect and biographies of all team members. And so, on 5 August, he contacted the University of Toronto: 'I understand that H&K have forwarded to you information for inclusion on a website relating to the 1918 influenza project. My name and CV were included in that package and I would like it removed.'

On 5 August, I wrote to the SAG: 'I, like you, have received the "final" version of the 1918 project press backgrounders. I place "final" in quotes, as (1) this was decided by H&K and not the SAG; and (2) H&K's actions of today make "final" untrue ... I have just received a fax from H&K, London, in which they state that I should send them the *"final"* draft to the Company in order that they can send the "final, final" changes to the University of Toronto.' I faxed Sian Wright yet again on the 5th: 'Please find attached the amendments, which were suggested by the SAG today. Please send me the final version of the press pack which you send to the University of Toronto.'

I was asked to send a fax to John Oxford and copy the letter to the SAG, after two SAG members complained of John's advertising our project on his website and telephone message system. I wrote, 'We have a serious problem, namely, unauthorized disclosure to the media. I addressed this issue with you in my letter of 27 July, 1998, as you had informed me that interviews were taking place. You simply cannot grant interviews ... I must ask you to delete your Company's telephone message, which says, "For further information on the 1918 project, please contact Professor John Oxford in writing." I must ask that you forward all requests to Professor Tom Bergan and myself. You cannot include project information on your Company's website without the approval of the SAG. I must, therefore, ask you to remove any reference to the project.'

Another Final Press Pack – Version A or Version B?

On 7 August, John Oxford suggested an alternative version to the 'final' document approved by the SAG. It (version A) omitted the 'offending' section on respect for the deceased, because, according to John, 'We all assume this anyway.' John explained that 'Version A also has telephone and e-mail addresses of the team in place.Version B includes the Section on "Respect" and has only the number of Kirsty Duncan and Tom Bergan.'

On 7 August, Sian Wright faxed the SAG: 'Professor Oxford and Sir John Skehel would like the SAG to vote on which text (Version A or B) should be submitted to U of T. Since they have expressed to us that they are unhappy with the text being submitted as it stands, we obviously cannot e-mail the text to U of T. This will, of course, mean that the SAG decide collectively and I regret that the matter of the text has not yet been resolved.' Before I could respond, however, I already had a fax from Tom (as Europe is hours ahead) to Sian Wright. 'Unfortunately, I have not had a chance to read the final text per se, but have faxed my answer regarding generalities (version A/B) to Professor Kirsty Duncan. This has partly practical reasons, as she is next to the website operator but also formally, since she – according to my recollection – would appear to be the only person to actually organize SAG voting.'

There was no point dealing with Sian Wright. She refused to respect my team's protocols. I telephoned Dr Martin Godfrey directly: 'You were so helpful to me the last time. I need your help again. I am furious by what's taken place today.'

'Kirsty, I'm sorry. We're in a very difficult position.'

'How? Your company made promises to me that you've broken.'

'We have bigger commitments to the Johns; we do the PR for ....' So that was it! At last I understood why H&K always looked to Sir John and John Oxford for approval. His voice trailed off, and he failed to finish his sentence. I jumped in, 'I beg your pardon?'

He ignored my question and instead asked, 'What do you need?'

'I want the text e-mailed to U of T as promised. I also want the section on respect and dignity, and I want only Tom and my name as the contact people.'

'Can you put that in writing to us so that people know we're acting on your orders?'

'Yes.'

After hanging up the phone, I quickly banged out a fax to Dr Godfrey: 'There is NO version A or B. Please send the text, which was promised to be sent yesterday. Again, there can be only contact details for Professor Tom Bergan and myself; we are the only two spokespersons for the team ... The section on respect and dignity must be included ... Finally, I require that the promised text be sent to the University of Toronto immediately. I require a fax confirming that this has been done.' I faxed the SAG members to let them know that the version to which they had made their amendments was sent to the University of Toronto. 'I understand that some of you are disappointed with the text ... It is very unfortunate that the relationship with H&K was difficult ... It is also very unfortunate that previous, private interests were used to influence the development of the document.'

Media Plan

While lengthy negotiations took place with H&K regarding the press pack, both Tom and I continued talking to the governor of Svalbard about our necessary media plan. The governor requested that Norwegian broadcasters and still photographers have access to the tent over the graves. Other members of the media, who were allowed at the cemetery, could then ask the Norwegians for film.

I knew that the SAG would not react favourably to the governor's ruling that the media have access to the tent. Rob Webster, John Skehel, and John Oxford all complained. I also knew that National Geographic would step aside if it could not have the same access as was earlier discussed.

On 17 July, following an angry phone call from John Oxford, I faxed him: 'Last week, I spoke personally to all the National Geographic people with whom I had been dealing. (H&K offered to talk to National Geographic. I refused their offer. I felt that I had to make the very difficult calls.) I explained that the Governor required that NRK (Norwegian broadcasters) and NTB (Norwegian still photographers) be the only people on site. I explained how sorry I was. National Geographic graciously bowed out. It is important to note that we are not the authority in Svalbard. The Governor is the authority. The Governor required that there be access to the tent. Tom softened this requirement by allowing photography to a depth of only a few centimetres from the surface.'

National Geographic on 17 July sent a pleasant and reassuring note. 'I know this has been a painful process for you. It's great to be able to make everyone happy, but you can't always do it. We're delighted that the science goes on!' The same day I heard from the governor's office: 'We refer to our telephone conversation, and confirm that NTB is the only photo team allowed in the tent to be erected above the Longyearbyen Church Yard ... NTB must as retribution use its distribution network and offer all editorial offices the photos according to the usual rules.' A further communication from the governor on the 17th read: 'We are happy that the research team will practise such an open policy towards the public as you have outlined in your letter. We are convinced that the access of NRK and NTB to inside the tent will make it easier for the public to understand this very special research. We accept that the research team decides from what point it is no more safe for a photo team to be inside the tent. Their limit has been set at 5 cm under the surface. It is up to the research team and NRK and NTB to agree en route when this is point is reached. Finally, we feel that it is a good idea to have press conferences at the hotel, up to daily."

After months of negotiating, the team had come up with an acceptable press package, suitable text for a web site, and a plan for dealing with the media that the governor of Svalbard approved. Thus we had met the final condition of my permission: 'A strategy for the handling of the Press and TV shall be made and submitted to the Governor for consideration as soon as possible and at least 6 weeks before the start of the excavation.'

Later, when the press packs arrived at the excavation site in Longyearbyen, most of the journalists had already left town. John Skehel's biography and photograph appeared in the press pack, although he had asked not to be included. A photo of Charles Smith served for both Charles and Tom. Tom, on hearing that Charles's face appeared beside the Norwegian co-ordinator's name, refused to let the press pack be released in Norway.

14 Money Wars

May–August 1998

NIH Funding?

We had reached the last important hurdle: funding for phase II, the exhumations. Roche had guaranteed funding, although the cheque had yet to arrive. Funding from the National Institutes of Health (NIH) was pending.

On 6 May, Rob Webster drafted a project update for SAG approval before sending the update to NIH. He wanted to explain the need for the Svalbard samples and hence for funding: 'The question can still be asked as to why we need additional information on the 1918 Spanish influenza virus when Dr. Jeffrey Taubenberger has already published a partial sequence and reportedly has an additional paraffin lung sample and tissues obtained from one sample in the permafrost in Alaska.' Webster offered seven possibilities: '(a) Providing sequence information on multiple samples of influenza virus from 1918 from a different geographical region. (b) Providing clues on the molecular basis of virulence of the virus. (c) Determining the extent of co-infection with other organisms. (d) We have the possibility of characterizing the sequence of other organisms present in the bodies. (e) The project is carefully planned to protect the environment and yield high quality samples. (f) We have the unlikely possibility of isolating and characterizing the 1918 virus. (g) The international community knows of the existence of these bodies so it is vitally important that this study is conducted by responsible scientists with approval of Norwegian authorities.' Once approved by the SAG, the update would be faxed to NIH, and the team would wait to hear about funding for the exhumations.

Funding Phase II

On 27 May, John Oxford faxed me to let me know that a number of us should obtain our funding from the NIH grant: 'It seems obvious that you, Charles, his assistant, and Tom should arrange your finances ... from the NIH grant.' Unfortunately, the team did not know yet if it had NIH funding.

Tom Bergan faxed John on the 29th: 'Does your letter to the effect that the Roche grant will not pay for me perhaps mean that my further project participation and/or presence at Svalbard is truncated?'

On 31 May, Tom broached the subject of funding again with Oxford. 'The problem with NIH is that so far there is no money from there. It does not make any difference to me what the source of fund is, of course (perhaps with my accent you feel I am American?), but without real money and not just prospects of such, the consequences might be as I felt.'

On 1 June, I approached John as well. 'Roche will have to cover our expenses. If NIH funding is renewed, we can repay the Roche grant. It is not possible for all team members to pay their own accommodation. All accommodation costs will have to be paid up front, as accommodation costs were paid the first time. There can be no question regarding funding for Les Davis or Peter Lewin. Both are valued members of the team ... Roche will have to cover their flights and accommodation. Could you please give me Torsten's [John's contact at Roche] phone number, as (1) I would like to thank him personally for the grant and (2) explain the difficulties in funding?'

John responded to me on 3 June: 'I feel we will all have to readjust to the orthodox manner of reclaiming airfares and accommodation after we have paid them from the forthcoming two grants.' To date, however, we had only one grant.

On 8 June, I faxed John again regarding funding. 'As Co-Principal Investigator on the Roche grant, I would very much like to have the opportunity to speak with Torsten. I would, therefore, be most grateful for Torsten's phone number. It is very important that you and I, as Co-Principal Investigators, both communicate with the granting agency. I would like to communicate the following to Torsten ... the need for up-front funding of flights and accommodation. (We are running short of time, and funding must be sorted out in order for me to book travel arrangements.)'

John answered me the next day: 'In essence we cannot pay everything from the Roche grant because we will not have enough cash ... it is quite proper for you, Charles and his colleague, and Tom to direct your claims from now on to Rob. I do not think it will help to have any extra person negotiating finance. Our problem is obviously a relatively minor cash flow issue.'

Minor Cash-Flow Issue

I wrote team members on 9 June to update them regarding the team's finances. 'It is with great regret that I must ask you to book your own flight to Oslo, as I had promised to undertake this job at the Toronto meeting. Unfortunately, funding cannot be provided in advance of travelling. Therefore, I cannot be responsible for booking (and paying) air fares. I sincerely hope that you understand. I apologize for any inconvenience.' On 15 June, I faxed Dean Sheila Cameron at the University of Windsor in order to request funding for my trip.

On 11 June, Tom told me 'I shall have to inform the governmental agencies about financial constraints which endanger the project as I will definitely not get involved in something that will harm my reputation and put me in personal debt. This is out of the question.' He faxed John Oxford on the same day. 'It seems that the finances are not in order. One thing that concerns me is whether I am being de facto exploited, to straighten things out here and to satisfy clauses that a Norwegian project participant is required by the Norwegian government. There is NOBODY here including hospital and university that would ever forward any money for the project. To think that they are happy to dish out money for their employees is tantamount to imagining things. I hope reimbursement for instructed travel is forthcoming very soon; a sum corresponding to two months of my pay is an unacceptable problem.'

On 13 June, Tom thanked John for a small cheque, owed to him for seven months; team members were to wait only fourteen days for reimbursements. Regardless, Tom was still owed 36,985 Norwegian crowns for travel to Toronto and London.

Both Tom and I were tiring of John's lack of co-operation in trying to sort out the team's finances. And so, on 13 June, we both faxed St Jude (Rob Webster's institution) for a copy of the NIH grant in the hopes that we could perhaps better organize funding. Neither of us ever received the requested document.

On 13 June, John Oxford faxed Tom. 'I am sorry about your late payment but £40 is not a world-shattering amount! More of a problem is your £3,600 for the Toronto meeting. At present, we have zero funds in the 1918 account ... Because of the lateness of settling the H&K decision QMW [John's institution] will not receive any cash flow until July.'

Tom had been out of pocket £3,600 for almost two months. And despite John's saying that Roche funding was not dependent on the team's committing itself to H&K, it appeared that 'the team's late acceptance' of the company had delayed the payment.

Tom followed up with John on the 15th: 'Your fax this afternoon was not good news. For one thing the huge amount of £3,600 is not only for Toronto, but also for London on 21 May 1998. It is very regrettable that one was led to believe that there was money for travel when there is none. It is inexcusable budgeting. I should have stayed here instead of going to Toronto and regret very much that I was even lured to increase the deficit further by going to London 2 weeks ago when it must have been even more apparent that no money was available. As you will surely understand, I have no way of paying myself, even temporarily. If there is no money, this project is dead and I must tell that to the Sysselmannen when I see them tomorrow. The project is hinged on solvency for whatever we undertake.'

Tom was absolutely right. I had been asking since the Toronto meeting for a detailed budget of the accounts. No budget was ever provided. At one point I did, however, see a draft budget, which showed that John had paid his staff £5,000 from the Roche grant for the 'administration' of the project. John was paying his staff with our joint research grant. When both Tom and I asked for an explanation, we were both ignored.

On 15 June, John faxed Tom: 'To put it mildly, there are some "local difficulties" as regards funding which are giving cause for serious alarm. These relate to our failure to date to execute the SAG decision to appoint H&K to take responsibility for PR.'

I faxed John on 16 June: 'I would be grateful if you could provide me with: (1) a list of the names of team members, who are currently owed money by the project; and (2) the amount of money owed to each team member. I require this information by Thursday. I now understand from yourself and others that there is no money left in the current Roche grant. '

We were in deep trouble. The first instalment of Roche money was apparently gone. The second amount had yet to arrive, and we still did not have a guarantee of NIH funding. And phase II was just two months away. On 17 June, I learned that everyone was owed money. John wrote, 'As regards finance, we are all owed something from the account at present. We are co-passengers in the same boat!' John did not appreciate what he considered harassment from Tom and me, and on 17 June he wrote to the whole research team. 'I have received some flak, mainly from Tom but also from Kirsty about delayed payment of invoices. Since Lars is my friend (still) I am used (sometimes) to irate telephone calls from Norway so I am not fazed by it! In fact I even support Norway in the World Cup! Finally, I would prefer not to be harassed about non-payment of small sums ... We do have permission to entertain on occasion (£40 per head approximately) and we are all allowed to charge alcohol with a meal, so there is some good news! Sorry for the little lecture but thought it would clear the air of any ill feeling, set the scene properly for future claims within our strict budget.'

On 17 June, I spoke with Tom: 'There is no forcing John to co-operate. I am so embarrassed by his not paying our colleagues ... I'm powerless. I have no way of fighting him. He holds the money ... You are powerless. It is not your fault. He is unscrupulous. You can't force him to do anything he doesn't want to do. He uses the money or lack of money to do things his way ... How can we get him to pay for everyone's accommodation and flights up front? Alan thinks that he is pulling the same thing that he did at phase I. That is, he is waiting to the last minute to "save the day" and be the "big hero." I don't think that is the case though. I think he really expects all of us to pay up front. I've explained that that is not possible.'

'Kirsty, you can't do anything ... I have one more thing to tell you. I will not go to Spitsbergen if John does not pay.'

'Tom, what do you want me to do? You know I can't force him.'

'Kirsty, I don't know what can be done. But, I'm telling you now. I won't go. I'm also telling you that it won't be your fault. I know you've tried.'

Having spoken to Tom, I again faxed my team. 'I would be grateful if you could send me an itemized list of any monies which you are currently owed by the project by this Friday (June 19th, 1998). I would very much like to know what is owing so that: (1) payment can be arranged; and (2) proper planning for phase II can take place ... This is an exciting time for the project! Many years of hard work and extensive planning for phase II are about to come to an end. This is the time for all of us to pull together and be supportive of one another's efforts.'

John faxed me on 18 June: 'As advised previously ... the claims can take anything from 6–8 weeks to be processed at this end.'

On 25 June, Tom faxed me: 'I am getting a bit saturated by "scud missiles" from John Oxford, and his lack of understanding that appropriate financial planning is essential for a project like this. Let me also state in writing that I have no intention of going to Spitsbergen in August if my flight tickets and hotel are not prepaid.'

On 26 June, I wrote to Webster and Oxford for a detailed spending account of phase I and a budget for phase II. There was some good news. Tom faxed John on 26 June. 'Today Peter called and said that you had sent him a note guaranteeing that funds would be sufficient for his travel.' John had finally agreed to fund Peter Lewin, one of the very first team members. Peter's medical training and his medical archaeology skills would be most useful.

John Oxford faxed Tom Bergan on 2 July, after discussing funding with Rob Webster. 'We will be utilising the conventional procedure for grants. All participants will pay individually by credit card or cash and then claim from either NIH or Roche.'

We had NIH funding! That was positive. However, neither Rob nor John seemed to appreciate what air fares and three-week hotel stays in Longyearbyen would cost.

Negative Account Balance

John faxed the SAG on 7 July regarding the team's finances. 'I have had several requests for a viewing of the 1918 account. It has deteriorated since you last saw the status in Toronto and it is now in the negative.' On July 9th, John faxed me the requested financial statement. I thanked him for the cash-flow statement, and requested further information: 'I would be grateful for a detailed accounting of the Retroscreen payment of £5000, since we are each obliged to submit detailed invoices for faxes, phone bills, etc. I would be grateful if your covering letter and cash flow statement could be faxed to the entire team ... Last, I am eagerly awaiting the budget for phase II.'

On 21 July, only three weeks before the excavation, I again requested a budget of John Oxford. On the 27th, I appealed to John: 'We have a real problem. I have heard from many team members that they simply cannot book their accommodation and flights on their credit cards. Moreover, their institutions will not cover their costs. What can be done? ... You said that "the beauty of the Roche grant was that it did not have to run like the NIH grant. The Roche grant even covered clothing." We cannot afford a change. Things are getting desperate. We leave very soon. The flights have to be paid in advance and the hotel must be paid 15 days after our stay.'

More trouble on the 28th. John was no longer paying for Peter. I faxed John as soon as I heard the latest from Peter: 'Again, Peter Lewin must go. I will not allow Peter to pay his own costs, as he has paid his own costs before. Moreover, you approved his trip; you said that we had the money.'

John faxed me back on the 29th: 'I am sorry about Peter Lewin but both Rob and I made it clear that we have to establish a budget *before* spending it! I am sure you will agree. I expect to have this today ... If we include Peter then we must save by curtailing days spent in Svalbard. Alternatively, he could pay his own fare?'

I called John immediately after receiving the fax. 'John,' I said, 'you can't leave Peter out [John and Rob were willing to pay for everyone except for Peter]. You can't make a promise, which you even put in writing, and then break it. It is not honest.'

'Well, there's no money.'

'John, if there is no money, it is your fault. You were looking after the money on behalf of the team.'

'Tom spent a whole whack of money by travelling first class.'

'John, please, Tom's flight did not break the bank. Mismanagement of funds did.'

'I don't like your attitude.'

'I don't really care, John. I just want a guarantee that Peter's trip will be paid for. He is a valued member of the team. He was involved long before you were.'

'Well, what do you want me to do?'

'You're going to have to find a way to cover Peter's expenses. And I don't care if that means your stay is reduced. You made a promise and you'll have to keep it.'

John faxed me. 'Obviously the situation is difficult with Peter, as Peter is a respected member of the team. It is just that we *do not have the cash* ... I expect Peter would be prepared to finance his fare and accommodation – after all it is an exciting trip. I will give him a ring.' I called Peter and warned him that John would be calling. Peter, always the gentleman, said, 'Kirsty, don't worry. I don't mind paying up front. I know how these things work. I am sure that I will be paid. You have enough to worry about. It's okay.'

Despite Peter's understanding, on the 27th, I faxed John: 'Peter Lewin has already booked his flight. You guaranteed Peter and me that he was going. You cannot, and must not, now turn around and decide otherwise. This is simply wrong and unacceptable.'

I faxed the team on 29 July to rally the troops. 'We are about three weeks away from phase II. This should be an exciting time. However, we have a number of issues which must be addressed immediately. The most important issue is pre-payment of fees ... Please find attached Professor Tom Bergan's letter regarding pre-payment.' The letter was addressed to the governor of Svalbard. It indicated that the project had financial troubles and that, as a result, Bergan could not be involved in the work. I continued: 'It is essential for Professor Bergan to be part of phase II, as: (1) he is the Responsible Medical Officer (RMO) for the expedition (the RMO is required by Norwegian law); (2) the Norwegian Co-ordinator is responsible for securing that the project is carried out according to the Governor of Svalbard's specifications; and (3) his involvement was a necessary condition for my being given permission to undertake the project. The work cannot go ahead without [his] involvement. We must cover his costs, and indeed every team member's costs, in order for the project to go ahead.'

There was no response. On 29 July, I again faxed the team after seeing Rob Webster's latest budget. 'Since we have shortened stays and eliminated stays there is room for further cut-backs. Removing H&K will save £1,500. A stay of 4 days for SAG members (outside of those directly involved in the work) would save an additional £960. The foregoing hardships can be overcome if we all pull together to work as a team, as we did in phase I.' H&K's stay was dropped.

As co–principal investigator on two grants, I had to be responsible for helping devise a budget. However, John and Rob chose to do it on their own. On 30 July, Tom faxed Rob: 'Another point is that your letter states that you, John Oxford, and Alan Heginbottom worked out costs. Since this whole project has Kirsty Duncan as team leader, she should have been part of the discussion. To the outside, including Norwegian authorities, she is responsible. Lack of economic control will be blamed on her, even though we, and a lengthy lawyer process, will explain what happened.'

On 31 July, I once again faxed all team members. 'There is need for concern with just over two weeks to the beginning of phase II ... The project is in jeopardy. In order for the project to continue, we must run phase II as we did phase I: that is, we must pre-pay phase II and we must use the Roche grant to pay back the NIH grant. However, there has been some good news. Professor Oxford has kindly agreed to cover some costs for one team member.' John had agreed to pay for some of Alan's costs, as he had the longest hotel stay. John and Rob had decided that the project leader did not need to be in Longyearbyen for the duration of the stay. 'If costs are to be covered for one team member, they must indeed be covered for all team members.'

Jeopardy

2 August. Tom called me early in the morning and explained that he would have to fax the governor his letter discussing funding. He was following through on his promise.

'Tom,' I said, 'before you send it, can I try one last thing?'

'What?'

'Perhaps I can explain to Roche's Noel Roberts that the project will die if John does not pre-pay your trip, as well as the other team members' trips.'

'Kirsty, I have to send it tomorrow. My name is at risk.'

I called Roberts. 'Hi, Noel. It's Kirsty Duncan. I hate to bother you at home, but I'm really in need of your help. I have in my hand a letter from Tom Bergan which he will fax to the Governor of Svalbard tomorrow if his trip to Longyearbyen is not paid in advance. Noel, this is very serious.'

'What does John Oxford have to say about this?'

I ignored his question. 'Noel, I have been asking for over two months for pre-payment of fares to avoid this situation. John is insisting that we all pay our own trips and get reimbursed later. He doesn't seem to understand that this is a hardship for most people.'

Noel, clearly annoyed, responded, 'I think Tom is being ridiculous. He should just pay. He is holding the team hostage.'

'Noel, the project is in the red, and John owes most of us money. Tom is afraid that if he goes, he will not be reimbursed ... Tom is especially afraid that the project will not be able to pay its bills in Longyearbyen ... Perhaps, you can talk to John. Noel, we're in real trouble.'

'I think you should be talking to Tom. His behaviour is beneath contempt.'

'Noel, there have been many complaints. People cannot afford to pay their flights and accommodation ... Please Noel, try to do something.'

'Kirsty, John is a friend.'

With Noel's last statement, I knew to expect nothing from him. I did know, however, to anticipate a letter from John. The expected fax came later that day. 'Just a quick request not to phone Noel – he is a personal friend and is on holiday and it just gives the impression that of the SAG, you and Tom are the only ones objecting to the NIH and QMW policy.'

John Oxford, John Skehel, and Rob Webster, who were staying only a few days in Longyearbyen, could afford to pay their stays. I was, however, staying almost three weeks, and Alan was staying even longer.

I was still no further ahead regarding pre-payment of Tom's trip. I had to talk to John one last time.

'John, I've got the letter in hand. Tom will fax it to the Governor tomorrow. Do you understand? The project is in real trouble.'

'He'll never do it. He's bluffing. He'll not risk the project. There's too much to gain personally and scientifically.'

'John, Tom is a well-known scientist. He doesn't need our project. Besides, the issue is not about personal gain or scientific gain; the issue is about his name being ruined by a project that cannot pay its bills. He has negotiated with the Norwegian authorities in good faith. He cannot risk having the project not pay its bills.'

'That's rubbish.'

'John, the project cannot go forward without Tom.'

'We don't need Tom.'

'I beg your pardon, John. No Tom, no project. He is both the Medically Responsible Officer and the Norwegian Co-ordinator. The project requires both. I have explained this in writing to you before.'

'Would anyone know if he wasn't present?'

'John, the team would know, and Norway would know. Tom needs to be present. How are you going to fix this?'

'It's not my responsibility.'

'It is. Now, how are you going to fix this?'

'I guess I could put his trip on my VISA card.'

'That would be excellent. I'll call Tom and let him know the good news. Thank you, John.'

I immediately called Tom and shared what had transpired. We would make it to Longyearbyen yet!

On 4 August, I faxed John. 'Again, thank you for kindly covering Tom's costs! Your great gesture is very much appreciated. I would be extremely grateful if a cheque could be brought to Longyearbyen for me. I have the second-longest stay (of the team members) and I have to cover my own costs.'

Rob Webster faxed Tom on 4 August: 'I am pleased to hear from Kirsty Duncan that your travel costs have been paid by John Oxford."

At last, on 5 August, I faxed Rob Webster and John Oxford: 'The University of Windsor has agreed to cover my flights from Toronto to Oslo and Oslo to Longyearbyen. The University will have to be repaid. Unfortunately, the University will not cover my accommodation costs. I have no way of paying £2,400.00.' This did not include almost three weeks of food costs in the Arctic!

By early August, a budget had finally been organized, and up-front funding had been provided for Alan and Tom. Unfortunately, the rest of the team, including me, would have to pay and reclaim the money later. I had, however, done my best to arrange pre-payment for my colleagues. The team was at last on its way to Longyearbyen!

Part Four

Exhumations

15   Face to Face

16 August–5 September 1998

Air Canada's 747 rocketed down the runway, the wheels lifted – and then the excitement and fear set in. The plane was roaring towards Frankfurt, the first stop on my last journey to Svalbard, which culminated six years of work and possibly an eighty-year mystery.

During the flight, while those around me slept, I thought about the science, I thought about finding the answers. And I thought about the miners. How would I feel when their coffins were opened after eighty years of undisturbed rest? And what if something went wrong? Everything had been planned to the last detail. Everything had been approved by the world's leading flu and biosafety experts and by the Norwegian state authorities. But still I was concerned. After all, the permission and the responsibility were mine alone.

After two days of travel, on 16 August 1998, I arrived in Longyear-byen, 960 km from the North Pole. I was greeted by the Svalbard authorities and then escorted to my hotel.

As I unpacked, there was a knocking at my hotel door. It was the press. The media were beginning their blitz. Perhaps I could just finish settling in. No, that would be impossible. They had a deadline. They not so gently reminded me that I was obliged to be open and available to the press. They had seen the letter requiring that our team grant open access to the media. They had done their homework. Maintaining a safe and scientific work environment, and maintaining the sanctity of the site, would be difficult with photographers, journalists, and film makers running about the cemetery.

As soon as the press left my hotel room, Alan, Tom and I made our way to the cemetery for an initial inspection. And as always, the visit was emotionally taxing. I was returning to the place where I had first made my pledge, which I must now honour.

Following the visit, the three of us met for dinner, one of the few times I sat down to dinner in the restaurant over my three-week stay. We discussed the next day's plans.

Early the next morning, Alan began recording everything that he could about the graves and environs of the seven miners. Roll after roll of Polaroid photographs. Detailed sketches, maps, and scale drawings. My permission required that on our departure there be no trace of our having been at the cemetery. The careful mapping of every rock, stone, and cobble would allow the site to be restored to its original condition after the exhumations.

While Alan made endless observations, Tom checked on the delivery of hydro, freight, and water services. And I began meeting with the interested parties in the community. Visits to the school, the church, the mine, and the University Courses on Svalbard (UNIS). Visits to friends, the people of Longyearbyen. And always the hardest visit for last: 'the family' – the family of the young man who froze to death several hundred metres from home and was buried in the cemetery in the same row as the miners. It was an awkward visit. I did my best to reassure the young man's mother that his grave would not be touched and that great care would be taken during the work. Words. Promises. Rhetoric. There was nothing that I could say to ease her pain, nothing I could say to allay her fears.

While I was making my rounds, workmen installed the site cabin, complete with refrigerator for storing the all-important tea fixings for Britain's Necropolis Company and a washroom that, I was reminded time after time, was not fit for a lady. The cabin would provide respite from the cold and wet and also, we hoped, relief from the media. How naïve. Little were we aware of the boom mikes that would pick up our every discussion. There would be no privacy.

Later in the day, the shipping containers, packed in England with 17 tonnes of supplies, were loaded onto a truck at the port of Longyearbyen and transported to the cemetery (Figures 8 and 9). The truck driver bluntly reminded me that I must do things right. He cautioned me that the cemetery was a graveyard, not a laboratory. He explained that most people supported the project. However, he did not favour it. He tried to control his anger. He was a friend of 'the family.' But when he could bottle his rage no longer, he blasted me: 'The project has hurt my friends. I want to protect them from any more pain.' That night, Tom, Alan, and I presented the history of the project, the GPR results,

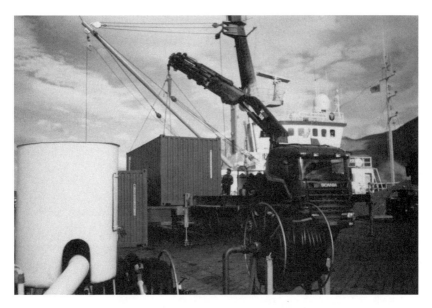

Figure 8   Loading equipment containers on to a truck at the port of Longyear-byen.

and the science of influenza to a press conference at the governor's office, at the request of the Norwegian authorities. The room was chockablock with reporters from the *New York Times*, the *Atlanta Journal Constitution*, and numerous Norwegian papers and with documentary teams from around the world. The roster also included journalist Esther Oxford, the daughter of John Oxford. Clearly – a conflict of interest for Esther.

The conflict, however, did not stop with Esther. John too was acting as a journalist; he was recording a radio documentary for the BBC. Prior to our trip, John had spoken to me of his 'unique opportunity' to make the documentary, and I had explained that it was illegal for him to record, according to the terms of our research agreement.

When the team asked John to stop recording in Longyearbyen, he made a 'grand display' of giving Esther the microphone and the tape recorder. Nevertheless, an American journalist later spotted him 'hiding in a ditch below the town secretly recording the team's activities.' (A few months later, Tom called me to say that he'd heard John's radio

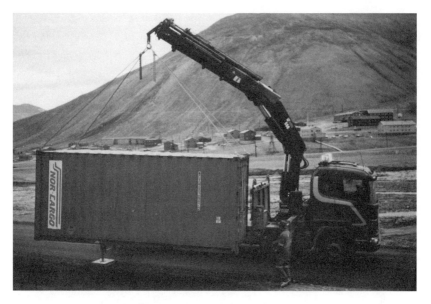

Figure 9   Receiving containers at the work site.

documentary, which had been broadcast throughout Europe and the United States. Tom was furious, as 'the documentary spoke of Professor Oxford and his project.')

At the press gathering, I presented gifts and letters from the University of Windsor, the University of Toronto, the city of Toronto, the city of Windsor, the province of Ontario, and Roy Cullen, a member of Parliament (Canada) to the governor of Svalbard thanking Norway for welcoming the scientists to Longyearbyen. From Mike Harris, premier of Ontario: 'On behalf of the Government of Ontario, I am pleased to extend greetings to the people of Longyearbyen, and to the Governor of Svalbard, the Honourable Madam Ann-Kristin Olsen. To the Ontario team working in Norway on a Project for the identification of the 1918 influenza, I offer my congratulations on the culmination of five years of intensive labour. My best wishes on the success of this cooperative endeavour.'

Following the conference, reporters requested interviews at the cemetery. I explained that I was uncomfortable with interviews there and declined their request. Perhaps we could talk here at the office. No, 'that would be no good.' They needed 'ambience.' Regardless, members of the governor's staff immediately ushered us off to the cemetery. We were even asked to smile.

After the last photograph at the cemetery, we were driven back to the hotel. It was after midnight.

The Necropolis team and Rod Daniels arrived in a Lear Jet the next day. Tremendous excitement. Flashing cameras, rolling film, a multitude of questions. Great attention on one of the Necropolis men. He was tattooed from head to toe: tattoos on his neck, on each of his fingers, and under his arms. Immediately he was judged. The journalists questioned his professionalism. They questioned his ability to do his work. They accused him of looking like a thug. However, this was the same man who later explained to me that people make 'a great fuss when someone dies, but, soon after, they forget the person.' When he works, he remembers 'that the corpses were once people with families,' and he often 'cradles 'em in me arms.'

Charles Smith and Barry Blenkinsop, his assistant, arrived the same day as the Lear Jet. Charles had been bumped to first class, as the airline was pleased to help a documentary film maker who was recording 'Charles's every move.' The film was to be part of a documentary regarding Charles's work as a pathologist 'as seen through the eyes of his young daughter.'

While the team members checked in at the hotel, Alan continued his slow, methodical recording. Towards dinnertime, he finished two days of observations of the seven graves. Necropolis and some of the scientists now wanted to begin unpacking supplies. However, I reminded them that we agreed that no work would be done until the team recognized those buried in the cemetery. The team would give thanks the following morning, and then the work would begin.

At night, all present team members gave a general lecture to UNIS. The members of the press were in full force and vocally disappointed when there was nothing new to report from the previous day.

Day 1. I had not been to bed. I couldn't sleep. Today was the day the work was to begin.

The Necropolis men, who perform exhumations for a living and understand the importance of saying 'thank you' to the families of those buried, arrived first. The scientists arrived haltingly; they objected, 'This is not science. They're dead.' But some families of the dead were still living in Longyearbyen. We, the invited guests, had to understand and respect the culture of our hosts.

Charles, who had slept in, rushed up the hill at two minutes to nine. He was still on Canadian time. We began. 'We are gathered to remember and honour the seven young men who died tragically in 1918, and indeed, all those buried in the cemetery.' I expressed the team's gratitude to the families of the miners for allowing us to undertake our work and to the people of Longyearbyen, Svalbard, and Norway. Finally, I ventured the hope that the team would succeed, and, in so doing, give thanks to the people of Norway.

Dr Smith led us in prayer, as Pastor Jan Hoifodt was away on holiday. Charles related that his grandfather Tobias Nelson (later called Bjorndahl) had left Norway to settle in Saskatchewan in the same year that Norway had achieved its independence from Sweden. He drew parallels between the lives of his grandfather and those of the seven young miners: both Bjorndahl and the miners had travelled to distant parts of the world to build a better life, and both had come to rest a great distance from their native Norway. He then spoke of visiting his grandfather's grave just a few weeks before his own trip to Norway. He noted that the cemetery in which his grandfather lay was well maintained, 'just like the cemetery in Svalbard.' He felt it a privilege to be a guest in Norway and to be a part of this special project. He regretted that Pastor Hoifodt was away, as he loved to hear him pray in Norwegian – the language of the heavens, according to his grandfather. Charles then apologized for speaking in English and prayed. They were beautiful, heartfelt words. A minute of silence in memory of the miners followed. Over the next two weeks, dozens of townspeople, in a town of just 1,200, said how much they had appreciated the tribute.

And then at last, work at the Svalbard cemetery officially began. Workers laid protective walkways of blue plastic matting, with vents to allow both sunlight and precipitation to permeate the ground and vegetation below, outside the cemetery fence (Figure 10). The team could leave behind no trace of its work. One misplaced foot could leave an indentation that would potentially mark the ground for a decade or more in the fragile Arctic environment. Next, the wrought-iron chain fence and posts that surrounded the cemetery were removed to ensure no damage to the protected, historical cemetery. Cheap, plastic perimeter fencing went up to safeguard the sacred site.

The six white crosses and the heavy tombstone that marked the

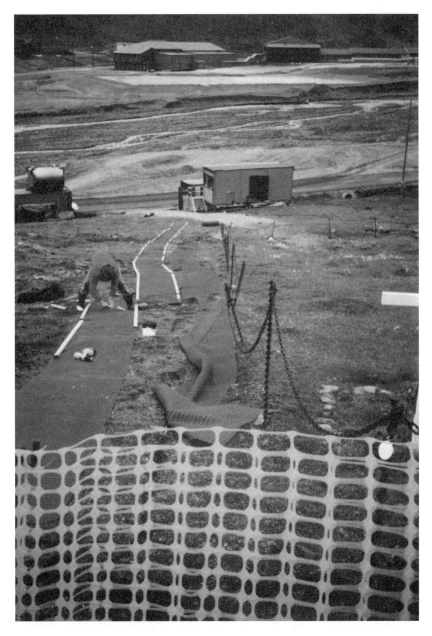

Figure 10   Laying protective walkways on the steep slope of the cemetery.

graves of the seven miners were then lifted from the ground, wrapped in burlap, and carried down the hill for safe storage (Figure 11). I left the cemetery. It was sad to see the dismantling of the beautiful church-yard.

Once the crosses were removed, workers installed the water tank, essential for the decontamination shower, and connected electrical power to the cabin and the work site.

Day 2. The heavy, back-breaking work commenced. Ten people hoisted two tents – one weighing a half-tonne and the other a quarter-tonne – up the valley side, which has a 1-in-4 slope. A considerable rise. Because the permission required that the team not use wheeled or tracked vehicles, the tents were raised by means of a hand-operated winch. It took over five hours to inch the two tents slowly up the steep hill (Figure 12).

Next, about 50 per cent of the equipment required for excavation was hauled by hand up the side of the valley: palettes to make a flat working surface, propane tanks for back-up power, and two-by-fours to build a soil-storage container. Cumulatively, some eight tonnes of materials went up the mountainside. We hauled load after load up to the site; as a result, I was honoured to be nicknamed 'The Iron Lady' by the Necropolis Company.

After the day's work, there was night watch to protect the site and supplies. Charles, who was still on Canadian time, kindly volunteered. I could not imagine anything more unpleasant. Barren, wind-swept, and dark. There would be no sleep, no warmth, and no protection. The only foods were 'powerbars' and 'powergels' – the energy foods of runners and triathletes – which the whole team was eating on a regular basis to keep warm and continue work. Powerbars were stuffed into every pocket. And if they began to freeze, they were quickly placed under our arms to thaw and then eaten. Although I was quite happy to work in the field all day, I secretly hoped that I would never have to pull night duty.

Day 3. The large tent was inflated. Up in 20 minutes! Six years to plan the work, and 20 minutes to inflate the mobile surgical unit, the type used to house the dead from airline disasters (Figure 13). The inflated tent was approximately 6.5 m by 5.0 m, with near-vertical walls. Its flat ceiling provided an inside working height of 2.5 m – necessary for the chemical decontamination shower.

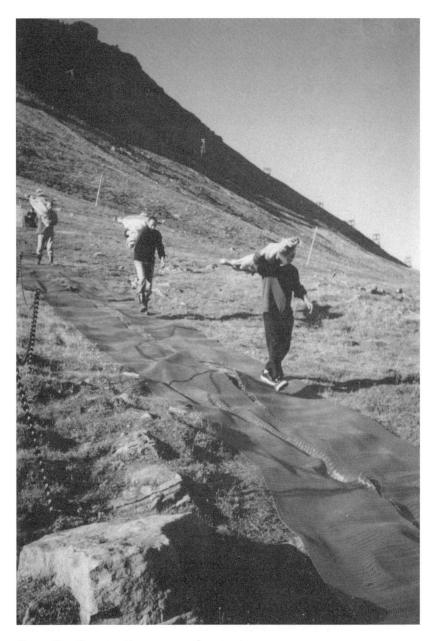

Figure 11   Carrying the grave markers to storage.

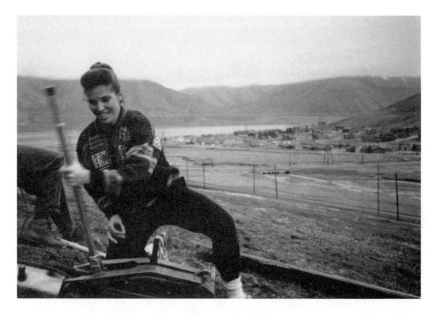

Figure 12   Kirsty Duncan winching the tent uphill.

Minutes later, the tent deflated, and our spirits with it. But then, 'Where's Charles?' Crawling on all fours, Charles emerged from the rapidly collapsing tent – a close call, a very close call.

After catching his breath, Charles politely inquired why the tent had deflated. Norske Hydro, which had strung long power cables to the site, had unfortunately run the main cable in front of the door of the outhouse. Someone tripped over the cable, pulled out a connector, and deflated the tent. The wiring was quickly sorted out, and the propane-powered generator and the remaining propane cylinders were hoisted into place using the hand-operated winch.

One of the highlights of my trip occurred during the day's lunchtime supply run into town. As Charles, Rod, and I travelled in our rented car, we stopped to meet a teacher, walking along the road, complete with rifle to protect her fifteen young students from polar bears. Charles and I went over to say 'hello' to the little girls. I asked them their names, ages, and grades. They gave few answers but giggled constantly. Their teacher asked them to talk to me in English. Their teacher must have explained the project to the children, because one little girl said to me, 'You work. And no more sickness.'

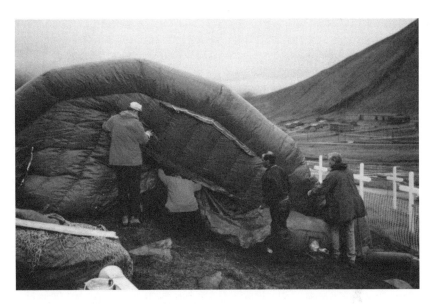

Figure 13   Inflating the mobile surgical tent.

Still keen to communicate with the children, I asked them if they had pets. Well, that was the magic question! They proceeded to shout out the kinds of pets they had: lizards, rabbits, piranhas, and parrots – exotic pets for a community that proudly boasts being home to Santa Claus. I then asked the girls if they wanted souvenir pins from Canada. They stretched out their hands, and their faces lit up. They shyly asked if they could have pins for the boys walking up ahead.

After our visit with the schoolchildren, Charles informed me that he was concerned about inadequate light levels in the tent, even though good lighting equipment had been shipped from England. Charles had been considering the use of fibre-optic lamps that surgeons wear when it occurred to him that miners use similar equipment. He suggested using mining helmets with their bright lights. But where to get such helmets? I needed to visit the director of Store Norske Spitsbergen Kulkompani, as I had not yet been able to deliver a thank-you gift to him. Charles, Rod, and I then went directly to the coal company. The director, after receiving his gift, casually asked how we would be lighting the tent. Charles explained his idea, and, in less than a minute, the director had arranged for mining hats and batteries to be delivered each day to the site.

Later in the afternoon we unpacked and inspected the medical supplies. The autopsy-sampling team practised donning and doffing special isolation apparel. The Martindale suits, or so-called space suits, had a large, clear, curved face plate with a filtered air supply that blew down over the wearer's face and upper body. The investigators also wore a thermal body suit, a tear-resistant suit of Tyvek, waterproof pants, several layers of hand protection (including puncture-resistant gloves), arm-sleeve protectors, full aprons, knee protectors, thermal socks, and rubber boots (Figure 14).

At last there was something for the media to shoot: a man in a green-and-yellow space suit. There would be no more of their sitting outside the work cabin and grumbling. Charles and Rod, who appeared as space man and trainer, were quickly surrounded – microphones above their heads, mikes by their waists, mikes at their feet. 'How does it feel? Is it easy to manoeuvre in?' No response. The questions were repeated. Charles continued to stand silent.

Rod then leaned into the giant face plate and carefully mouthed the questions to Charles. Charles, shaking his head and tapping near his ears, indicated that he could hear nothing. Problem number one: it was impossible to hear over the blowing air. Charles and Rod would need to use hand signals in the tent. Problem number two: Charles was freezing, despite wearing a thermal body suit. He would require more layers to protect him from the cold, blowing air.

While the media circus watched trainer and astronaut, ground-protection work continued inside and around the main tent. The tent floor and soil-storage areas were built to protect the surface layer of the tundra.

Night watch. Another lucky volunteer. Fortunately, not I. However, I was subject to another nighttime duty. After returning to the hotel from the field, I was handed a stack of pink slips requesting that I return the barrage of calls from the world's press.

I went immediately to my room, missing dinner in the restaurant with my colleagues. The managerial staff at the hotel voluntarily brought dinner to my room at about eleven p.m. Delivery of dinner would be repeated almost nightly for the remainder of my stay.

Day 4. Construction continued. Transportation of supplies continued. John Oxford and Noel Roberts arrived.

I placed a wreath outside the tent at the start of the morning's work to show our host community that we recognized the site as a cemetery,

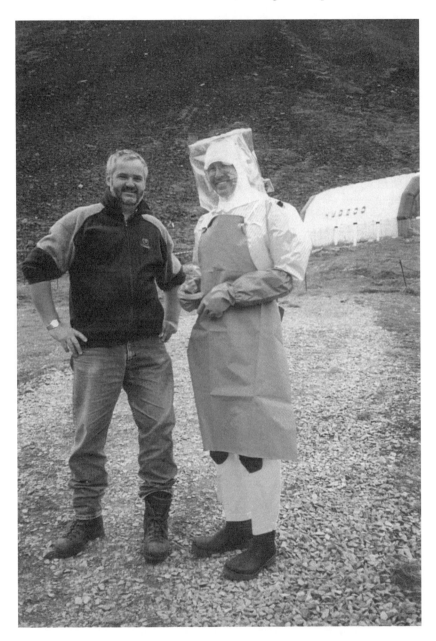

Figure 14   Charles Smith sporting the Martindale suit for Rod Daniels.

not merely as a workplace. The wreath was 'sending the wrong message,' according to Tom. 'The Project is about science. Moreover, a wreath is not laid at a work site.' Tom requested that the wreath be laid at the completion of our work. I agreed to the timing.

Later in the day, one of the Necropolis crew came to speak with me. He explained that Necropolis never begins digging until the graves have been blessed. The man was close to tears, as he did not think that the scientific team would observe Necropolis's tradition. The blessing of the graves seemed appropriate, and I approached Tom about having Pastor Hoifodt bless the graves.

Charles, Mark (the representative from Necropolis), Tom, his wife, Bodil, and I went to the church. Charles explained that the benison was a Necropolis tradition and that the pastor would honour the Necropolis workers and grant them peace if he would agree to their request. He kindly did so.

Back at the cemetery, a French documentary film maker said that she didn't know how I took some of the scientists' 'complaining, their attitudes.' I said only that I was exhausted and that I had had little sleep. She kindly asked if I was still willing to do the promised interview the next day. I said 'yes.' She said that she and her crew wanted to give me a break. Would I be available to go on a long hike up the glacier above the town? A respite from the work. I said 'yes' and thanked her for her kindness.

Late in the afternoon, Pastor Hoifodt paid a formal visit to the cemetery, as requested (Figure 15). he offered a Christian perspective on the relevant ethical and moral issues of disturbing a cemetery and then indicated why this research project must continue. He said that if the men knew that their bodies held the key to such a terrible plague, they would say, 'Of course, take samples of my body for research.' He read from the Bible and then led us in prayer (Figure 16). He then entered the protective tent and initiated the digging by removing the first piece of tundra that covered the graves of the seven miners.

Workers from the Necropolis Company removed sections of the ground cover and placed them like parts of a giant jigsaw puzzle on a large receiving platform. The workers stored the transposed tundra carefully so that each piece could later be returned to its original position.

Night watch: Keith, a Necropolis worker, was the unlucky volunteer. No one wanted the duty, since gale-force winds and freezing rain shook the cabin, and sleep-deprived guards imagined stalking bears.

The team's preoccupation with ice bears stemmed from Alan's regal-

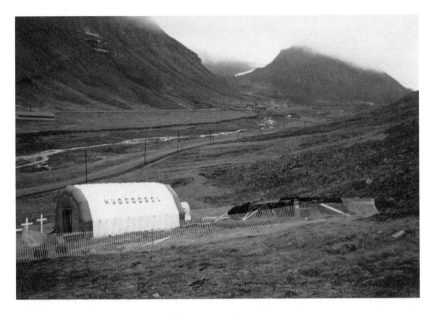

Figure 15   The work site, showing the surgical tent, perimeter fencing, and soil container.

ing everyone with nightmarish polar-bear stories. He had two favourites. The first: a colleague, who was rolled up in a brown sleeping bag on a beach, was mistaken for a seal by a polar bear, who then tried to make a meal of him. The second: a friend, asleep in his tent, was dragged out head-first by a polar bear. Apparently, said Alan, the bear wanted to play. After the appropriate gasps, Alan revealed that the men had luckily survived.

As if Alan's stories were not enough, Longyearbyen had many of its own tales. Jan Haugaland, director of the Norse Polar Institute and a world-renowned Arctic and Antarctic explorer, told me of his friend who was taking a group of boy scouts up on the glacier above the town. The friend was not going to take a rifle, but Jan convinced him to do so. When the leader and his group reached the top of the glacier, they were met not by one, but by two polar bears.

That night, while Keith was on duty, he heard a heavy battering against the cabin walls. And with thoughts of polar bears, he stepped outside to be frightened by, and to frighten ... two startled reindeer.

Day 5. Sunday morning, and some of the team attended the worship

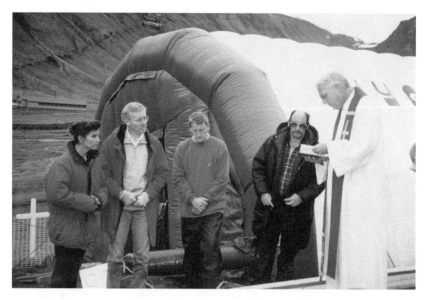

Figure 16   Pastor Jan Hoifodt blessing the graves.

service at the Norwegian Lutheran church. The pastor kindly conducted part of the service in English and asked Charles to read a pas-
sage in English from the scriptures with Dr Anders Christiansen, the
surgeon from Longyearbyen Hospital. Charles was elated.

While Charles spoke, I had a visit from a toddler, whom I had seen
wrapped in his mother's arms the previous year. He brought me a
hymn book. 'Thank you, sweetheart,' I said with a smile. This elicited
another hymn book. 'Ta.' And the third time, an armful of books. Back
and forth he scurried. When he finally ran out of books, he pinched
one from the nearest member of the congregation, who gently ended
the game. After the service we enjoyed coffee with the town's residents
in the church's fellowship hall, furnished with stuffed polar bears.

Following the service, Esther Oxford, who was gradually interviewing all team members, asked to interview me. The team was very concerned about her coverage of the project, as it was clear that her father
had discussed confidential team business with her.

One of her first questions to me was about leadership of the project.
She said that she had understood that the project was her father's.
However, since coming to Longyearbyen, she realized that the project

was clearly mine. I felt very sad for her. Despite her understanding, she would tell her father's guests (including my husband and me) in London a year later that she 'was biased from the beginning' regarding the writing of her story. She 'was determined to see Father succeed at any cost.'

She next asked about her father's role in the project. I was relieved that she had already asked Tom the same question. I gave the same answer as he had. 'Your father found Necropolis, and he found funding.' She asked what else he had done. I didn't answer. I was not about to tell her that her father had made life very difficult for many members of the team and that her father's budgeting had almost ended the project.

She then asked about my first meeting with her father. I talked about his enthusiasm and our similar interests in art and dance. In retrospect, however, I see the first meeting very differently today. John had volunteered to give his archival tissue samples to the team, and he asked in return that he and Rod be made part of the project. He never made good on his promise.

Esther next asked why Professor Lars Haaheim and CDC had pulled out of the project. I answered simply that according to their letter of 27 June 1997 they no longer had 'the necessary time and money to devote to the project.' 'But why did they really pull out?' she asked. I said, 'I can only go by what they communicated.'

It was a short interview. Esther asked about my personal life. I explained that my private business was not relevant to the project. She agreed. Nevertheless, personal details, gleaned elsewhere, would later appear near the beginning of Esther's multi-page article on the inner workings of the team, coloured by her father's comments.

The interview concluded with my saying what a difficult position Esther was in; she, however, said that she had her father's characteristics and she liked her position. She was, in her own words, her 'father's daughter.'

When we completed the interview, the French film makers took me on the promised glacier walk. We stopped briefly for our tour guide, rifles, and flares – protection against the ice bears. And then the long walk up the valley floor. During the hike, we crossed several meltwater channels draining away from the glacier, laying down ladders to traverse the raging, mud-filled rivers. And then we continued up the long, muddy moraine deposited at the snout of the glacier. At the top of the deposit, we strapped on our crampons and took our first tentative steps onto the glacier. And although it was breathtakingly beautiful, I could not help thinking of Jan Haugaland's story of the boy scouts and the two bears on this very glacier.

As the temperature plummeted through the afternoon, I thought of all the information that glaciers can tell us about past climate. Individual bands of ice, preserved over the last 10,000 years, give scientists an annual record of temperature and precipitation. Air bubbles trapped in the ice provide information about the composition of Earth's atmosphere over the last two million years. And acid spikes in the ice tell of past volcanic eruptions.

Then I remembered my team – slogging in the cemetery. I had to get back. The outing had been amazing. I had worn crampons, had walked on a glacier for the first time in my life, and had drunk the purest, freshest, coldest water atop the ice.

During the afternoon, the –70°C freezer to store tissue samples was winched up the hill and positioned in the protective tent. Electrical lines were installed, and medical supplies organized.

Outside the tent, the Necropolis team removed and stored the last of the tundra covering the seven graves. Construction was completed on the large container that would serve as a storage site for the soil, rock, and permafrost that would be removed from above the coffins. Digging of the permafrost began.

Day 6. Tom Bergan departed for Oslo, and Bjorn Berdal arrived to serve as the team's medically responsible officer (MRO). As on previous days, the members of the scientific team and Necropolis worked side by side, sharing in the various tasks from construction to site supervision.

The team played host to many visitors: workers from the community, curious schoolchildren, students from UNIS, timid reindeer, and beautiful Arctic foxes. We enjoyed a very special visit from school teacher Liv Arneson, the first woman to ski to the South Pole. She skied for 50 days hauling hundreds of kilos of supplies 1,200 km to the Pole. To train for her expedition, she first skied across Greenland. She then spent three months hiking through her neighbourhood in Oslo while carrying a 15-kg-backpack and 'dragging a bunch of old car tires along the ground' behind her. She inspired me with her determination, her will power, and her physical and emotional strength.

Rod struck a wooden surface while digging late in the afternoon. Charles and Alan immediately drove to the hotel to find me, as I had been working with the governor's office and the media, trying to sort out various documentary makers' disputes with Elliot Halpern and his film crew.

I longed to concentrate on just the work at the cemetery, but I had to liaise with the governor's office, the community, and the media. I had to make sure that everything was running properly and was being carried out according to our team's promises and our guidelines. Charles and I had an agreement. If ever he thought that the work was proceeding unsafely or unwisely, he would tell me, and I would pull the plug on the project. It was comforting to have someone beside me who put safety and 'doing the right thing' above everything else.

Now Charles and Alan told me breathlessly that Rod might have found the first coffin. At that point, however, all they had was a wooden surface. I knew immediately that the box was close to the surface, since Necropolis had been digging only a short time. We drove back to the site while Charles relayed more news. John and Gillian Oxford had been digging in the tent. I was furious. Only Necropolis was to have been digging. We had given detailed safety protocols to the authorities. Only the minimum number of people were to be allowed in the tent – only those required to be there. John should not have been inside. Gillian, who was not even a team member, clearly should not have been present.

We were about to learn what lay beneath the crosses. The team held a meeting in the work cabin, while the press huddled outside. My first duty was to transfer the supervisory role from Alan to Charles, because the work was progressing from excavation to exhumation. Charles then set in place a reduced work team, which went up to the tent in order to investigate whether or not the wooden surface was a coffin. The rest of us stayed down in the cabin. Those in the tent communicated with me via radio.

And those in the cabin waited with bated breath. After a few short minutes, we learned that the wood was indeed a coffin. Shortly thereafter, two other coffins were found. The three coffins were approximately 0.5 m from the surface, in the active layer of the permafrost. The day's work was finished.

Night watch. Charles had again volunteered for overnight sentry duty. The weather was stormy – grey sky, freezing drizzle, and gusting winds. The fear of polar bears was strong – and this time, for good reason. The coffins' contents were emitting a sweet, sickly stench.

Charles was concerned that the odour of decaying flesh would attract bears.

Alan, who had been to the Arctic season after season, assured everyone that polar bears were 'not likely to come this far from the water at this time of year.' He also cautioned us that since the cabin would be useless against a bear, we should run into the steel shipping containers if confronted.

About midnight, Charles received visitors. He welcomed the governor and two other government officials, who arrived to learn of the day's work.

Day 7. A fourth coffin was located early in the morning. I was extremely excited. We had actually found caskets. According to the media, however, I should have been devastated, since the coffins had been found in shallow ground. Remember Smith's first rule of exhumation, 'You don't know what you have until you actually do the work.' I had been prepared that we might find nothing, despite the historical, archaeological, and radar evidence. The team had been ready for many eventualities: bodies in coffins, bodies in shrouds, commingling of bodies, bodies buried shallowly, and so on. The media also suggested that the expedition was a great failure. We had not even unearthed seven coffins. Nor had we begun to investigate their contents. We had only four coffins. The team did not know if these were the coffins of the seven victims. And no coffin had been opened; only a small portion of the upper surface of each coffin had been exposed.

Nonetheless, the team was excited – except for John, who derided the project to members of the media who would listen to him. Rob Webster had just arrived from the United States. He greeted me with a big hug; he could barely contain himself. I told him that we had found coffins; I explained that they were more shallow than we had expected. He responded: 'This is science. We asked a question and now we are getting answers. This is very exciting.'

While Necropolis dug, Charles and Bjorn met with the director of Longyearbyen Hospital to ensure that the hospital's backup medical systems were ready should they be required.

The team's safety protocols recommended that those in the tent take an experimental drug to counter the influenza virus, should they be exposed to it. Only one Necropolis worker, Mark, took the drug. Unfortunately, he did not read the statement (enclosed with the drug) explaining that about 15 per cent of people who take the drug suffer significant side effects, such as severe nausea and vomiting. The poor man was among the 15 per cent, and had to be taken to the hospital.

While Mark recovered, the rest of the Necropolis team continued digging and soon exposed the remaining coffins – a fifth, a sixth, and finally a seventh. The men then dug beyond the seven coffins to confirm that there were indeed only seven.

It appeared that the seven coffins were those of the miners. It also seemeed that they were in the active layer of the permafrost. And although they would have been exposed to freezing and thawing since interment, they would have remained completely frozen 10–11 months per year over the last eight decades.

After we held the morning's press conference, Peter Lewin arrived. Peter would later prove invaluable when a young Necropolis man began coughing up blood and had to be taken to hospital. Immediate concern – the man had been digging in the ground and was now bringing up blood. Peter, calm and gentle, along with the staff of Longyearbyen Hospital, reassured the man at his hospital bed that his temporary illness was caused by 'too much of the Norwegian spirit.' A few days' respite from night life and the man recovered.

In addition to having excellent medical skills, Peter, always goodnatured and friendly, had a unique way of releasing team tension. We needed him. John was now openly discussing our findings with the media, despite our agreement that we communicate new findings only at the morning press conferences. Moreover, John had invited, without telling the team, two men from his medical school to the exhumations. It was apparent that they hoped to get samples from our work. I wouldn't be able to get samples back to Norway and Canada, but these interlopers requested samples for their medical school. After I introduced myself as the project leader, the two men stood motionless, staring at me – clearly confused by what I had said. They were barred from the tent.

After the seventh coffin was uncovered, John immediately informed the press that there were seven coffins and that the project was 'a bust' because the coffins contained only bones. Premature, surely. No coffins had been opened. Charles, supervisor for the exhumation, requested that John maintain silence. John ignored the request.

Charles and I were walking down the hill behind John later in the day when we both heard him say, 'This is dangerous. We could all go home in coffins' – in front of the Danish TV crew. Again Charles confronted John, who said that he was talking about the blue matting of the protective walkways, as the path was slippery. Our guiding principle for the project was safety. John's off-the-cuff comment could have shut down the project. The Danish crew kindly agreed not to use his remark.

Charles, after consulting other members of the team, particularly key virologists, banned John from the tent. John, unaware that I was at a meeting at the governor's office during the making of the decision, assumed that I was the instigator – calling me 'a megalomaniac and a control freak.' I was, according to John, 'not the easiest person in the world to get along with,' while he was 'a mild-mannered man.'[1] Charles had agonized over his decision to ban John. The decision was difficult for everyone. But it was also agreed that it was the right one; we could afford no more irresponsible remarks.

Late in day 7, it was decided to open coffin no. 6, since its lid was in the best state of preservation. I disagreed with the decision because I believed that the microenvironmental conditions surrounding coffin no. 6, particularly moisture, were poor for preservation of material. If any coffins were to yield material, I thought that no. 1 was likely to provide the best opportunity. Despite my training in both archaeology and environmental science, the virologists were not convinced. They felt that there was an urgent need to begin sampling the bodies (if indeed there were bodies) before they warmed up.

Sir John, former director of the WHO Influenza Centre, called a team meeting to discuss safety. He reasoned that the risk of finding live virus was even lower than 10^{-18}, as the coffins had been found in the active layer of the permafrost. He suggested that we could modify a number of our safety protocols.

He and Charles would allow the team inside the tent – except, of course, John. I had never expected to be present for the exhumations, according to our safety protocols. And although it would have been disappointing for me not to be present, safety had to come first. But as a result of the new protocols, I would be there with the young victims to convey my personal thanks.

Citizens and media alike asked why I felt so strongly about being beside the miners. From the media: 'Why the attachment? They're just bodies. They're old.' My response: 'Many people feel uncomfortable when a newly buried body is disturbed. They feel less uncomfortable when an older corpse is exhumed; the deceased appears less connected to the human world, as often there are no relatives to speak for him. At what moment in time does this dichotomy develop?

The media compared the victims to organ donors. Many people, they said, want to fill out organ donor cards in order to make a difference to another life. I said that we have the freedom to make our own decision regarding organ donation and the freedom to sign donor cards. I explained that the living relatives of the miners spoke for their dead kin. I hoped that had the miners themselves been given a choice, they would have agreed to the work. (During the digging, the earth too yielded up a remnant from two summers ago: a long-stemmed, faded yellow rose.)

Sir John, after discussing the safety issue, also brought up the sticky question of the laboratories. He said that the team did not need my lawyer's drafted lab agreement, which assured that all signing parties would receive samples and prevented a signatory from releasing results without the approval of all team members. Through experience, I knew that we needed the agreement.

It was already agreed that the samples had to go to the NIMR in London. But how were the samples to be divided? Earlier the team had agreed that they would be divided in the field.[2, 3] Now Sir John was changing the game. He argued that it would be easier and safer to divide them in the laboratory. He was contradicting himself. On the one hand, he was saying that since there was virtually no safety risk we could all be present in the tent. On the other hand, he was saying that it was safer to divide the samples in the lab, lest there be a safety risk. Nevertheless, Sir John convinced the team to divide the samples in his NIMR lab.

He then gave the team his word that once the samples had been tested for live virus and deemed safe, they would be shipped to Canada and Norway. I borrowed John Oxford's phone to put a call through to Tom, the Norwegian co-ordinator, the man responsible for returning the samples to Norway. Tom agreed with the decision. What choice did we have? There was no other BSL 4 lab available. And Sir John refused to sign the laboratory agreement. Our hands were tied.

After the team's discussion of safety, Mark cut into the lid and removed the three narrow, tongue-and-groove pine boards that formed the top of the coffin. Charles and Barry lay on opposite sides of the coffin, poised to begin the autopsy, while Rob and Rod stood by the freezer, ready to receive, label, and bag the samples. And I stood, pen in hand, ready to record the findings.

And then from the darkness of the pit – a corpse. 'Light!' called Charles. Peter illuminated the pit from above. A body lay bathed in the glow of a miner's lantern.

A multitude of feelings. I had waited six long years for this moment. I had feared this moment, and I was responsible for this awakening. But perhaps this man of nearly a century ago would reveal his story, his fight against the virus. And I felt sorry – sorry for the surviving families.

The body was exposed only from his hips upward. The team did not remove the rocks and dirt covering the lower half of the coffin, as the team was doing its best to limit the disturbance to the coffin, the grave, and the cemetery as a whole.

However, soon came the water, saturating the ground, and making it vulnerable to collapsing. From a climatological point of view, the year of our digging, 1998, was as unusual as 1918. Temperature records, which extend back to 1912 for Longyearbyen, show 1918 as one of the coldest years. The extremely low temperature was important, because the bodies would have frozen in a few days prior to their burial. One of the warmest summers on record was 1998. Warm conditions and an unusual amount of precipitation were melting the permafrost deeper and faster than usual. Because the active layer was saturated with freezing water, the ground became unstable.

Despite the icy water, Charles and Barry described the man of eighty years ago. No identifying marks. The body had not been clothed at the time of burial nor placed in a shroud. Instead, it had been wrapped in newspaper. We carefully examined all fragments of the wet paper hoping to find a date that would confirm that the body was a Spanish flu victim. Unfortunately, we found no date.

I did not and do not share the details regarding the appearance of the bodies, as there are family members of the miners still living. The body was, however, largely skeletonized. Despite this fact, the team did get good soft tissue samples, particularly of the brain. A total of thirty-eight samples was recovered from the one body; the tissues were packed, labelled, and stored in the freezer.

The autopsy had started at 4:30 p.m. and had finished at 7:00 p.m. The coffin was then reconstructed, and the young man was once again laid to rest – never to be disturbed again, we hoped. I gave my thanks.

The team left the tent exhausted but in high spirits, only to walk past a dejected John Oxford, who was keeping a vigil at the cabin with the rest of the media. But as Charles reminded me, 'Kirsty, it was a group decision. It is for the best.' John's activities provoked his virologist colleagues to complain, 'We tried to warn you about him – his reputation proceeds him wherever he goes.'

We all went to dinner back at the hotel restaurant. What a delightful change from dinner alone in my hotel room.

At eleven p.m., the team met to plan the activities of the next day and the morning's press conference. A Necropolis man, speaking from experience, said that he did not think that we had reached the Spanish flu victims and that the seven miners we sought were perhaps buried deeper in the permafrost. He said that the coffins were of German design. He guessed that the bodies that we found could have been buried when German ships destroyed Longyearbyen: the easiest way to hide war atrocities 'was to bury the dead on top of other bodies in the cemetery.'

The scientific team had great respect for the Necropolis men. We decided that we should look deeper into the permafrost. I argued that seven coffins had been found below seven markers and were probably our seven miners.

John had left the room and was not present when we discussed the Necropolis man's hypothesis of war dead. (Despite his absence, he later provided for publication the same detailed account of hiding war atrocities.[1] Someone had clearly leaked information to John, who was to have no private information that he could relay to the media.) He later returned to the meeting room, left before the session ended, and was overheard telling his wife and the media what the team was doing the next day.

Day 8. The excavation was extended to the right of the coffins down to the frozen ground (1.5 m) and under coffin no. 7 in order to determine if there was a lower row of coffins, as radar images and Necropolis suggested. The team was first encouraged by Necropolis's finding of what appeared to be a capping stone, placed over victims of infectious disease in the hope that the infection could not spread through the rock.

The men increased their pace. They took turns hammering, shovelling, bucketing out, and wheeling the melting permafrost to the storage tank. It was difficult work. They could tolerate being in the hole only about 10 minutes because the wet slush was so chilling. Despite their strenuous effort, the Necropolis workers did not find a lower layer of coffins.

We held a team meeting at eight p.m. Should we begin removing the tissue samples from the bodies, or should we penetrate deeper into the permafrost? Everyone except for me wanted to continue looking deeper. I was concerned about the safety of the men; working conditions were becoming more and more difficult. I was also worried about the rising water's damaging the cemetery and the increasing threat of the pit's collapsing through ground slumping. Charles assured me of the men's safety and of the pit's integrity. The team agreed to go ahead with the sampling of the other five bodies the next day. Digging would commence the day after that to find deeper coffins.

At nine p.m., Bjorn, Charles, Sir John, and I went for dinner to the home of Jan Haugaland, director of the Norse Polar Institute. Jan's wife, Anna, prepared a reindeer stew, salad, and cheesecake. Jan regaled us all with his tales of adventure at both Poles, where he had led numerous expeditions.

Day 9. This was, at last, a day of rest for the excavation team, which had worked extremely hard digging into the permafrost and had not had a day of rest since arriving. Digging with jackhammers and picks in permafrost was akin to digging in concrete. It was back-breaking, bone-chilling work. Ten minutes in the pit. Change hands. Ten minutes in the tent. Switch. Eight gruelling hours a day, while freezing water soaked the pit and numbed the workers' feet.

Despite the horrific conditions, three of the scientists were willing to help with the drilling because they were accustomed to physical labour. Both Charles and Rod enjoy working with their hands; Charles, on his farm, and Rod, in restoring his home. Rob, seemingly unaware of the cold, enjoyed operating the jackhammer. He was excited about everything – the physical work, the science, and the Arctic. He eagerly took turn after turn in the pit.

While Necropolis rested, the team opened the five remaining coffins, as we had permission to examine only six of the seven coffins. It was a special day for all of us. In fact, Charles privately told me that 27 August marked 'the highlight of [his] medical career.'

Aware of Necropolis's concerns, Charles and Barry spent a long time examining the ribs and the vertebral column of the dead in order to assure that there were no bullet marks from execution-style shootings. And while sampling was taking place in the tent, Necropolis faxed Alan's drawing of the coffins to Service Corporation International (SCI) in London to determine whether or not the coffin was of Norwegian design. It also faxed the drawing to SCI in Oslo, which started analysing the evidence. By our evening meeting, we knew that the coffins were of Norwegian manufacture and that that type had been in production from about 1910 to 1960.

The governor had given us permission to perform autopsies.

The autopsy of corpse no. 1: Sir John assisted Barry Blenkinsop with the autopsy, which was hard, cold, and physically demanding. Everyone waited anxiously as the lid was opened. The tissues in coffin no. 1 were in much better shape than those of coffin no. 6, as I had suspected, because the ground conditions were much drier. Rod and Rob labelled, catalogued, and stored the samples. I maintained the lighting.

Next, coffin no. 2 was examined. Rob assisted, having taken over from Sir John. No one spoke. The atmosphere was tense. More good samples from major organs. We skipped no. 3, since we agreed that it contained the man whose body we were not allowed to disturb.

Charles assisted Barry with coffin no. 4 and then asked me to assist with coffin no. 5. I was thrilled and very nervous. My academic background includes anthropology. I was finally going to have the opportunity to practise what I had learned. I had only a second to think before descending into the pit. My thoughts were of my first laboratory courses in osteology and palaeopathology, in which the professor carefully explained that all bones were to be handled with extreme care. She explained that many of the bones in the lab came from India and that people often sold their bodies in order to pay for life's necessities. The sales entailed great sacrifice, since religion dictated that the ashes of the faithful be scattered in the Ganges. I recalled the lesson in responsibility and then entered the pit.

After the samples from coffin no. 6 were carefully stored in the freezer, Charles questioned whether to continue sampling at coffin no. 7. He was not sure if it was safe to work in the pit; the water was continuing to rise, and a cave-in was becoming an increasing and ever-present threat. Eventually he decided on sampling.

Rod assisted Barry with the autopsy of coffin no. 7. In examining the last sample, Rod noticed a fragment of newspaper. He read the faded scrap's lettering, then the figures, '1 ... 9 ... 1 ... 7.' He then repeated, '1, 9, 17. We got them." Everyone repeated, '1, 9, 1, 7.' The solemn atmosphere of the tent erupted in complete and utter jubilation. We knew that, with only a few ships visiting Longyearbyen each year, newspapers would have been kept for long periods of time. We were now virtually sure that the newspaper wrapped our long-sought victims.

The sampling was at last finished. Over 100 samples were labelled and stored in the freezer. The expedition had been a great success – we had accomplished our goal, to retrieve soft tissue from the victims.

Under Charles and Sir John's strict orders, we were not to discuss the exciting finds with John, who was patiently waiting at the bottom of the hill. While John waited with the media, Alan spent the day poring over the GPR data, trying to understand why the radar had shown disturbance to a depth of ~2.0 m, although the coffins were found at 0.5 m. Two theories emerged. Alan and Barry suggested that the community dynamited the permafrost to produce a burial pit – as it did in later decades. The use of explosives would explain the disturbance to a depth of ~2.0 m. Barry further proposed that the community was probably so afraid of the killer flu that it did not take time to remove the dynamited soil from the pit. Instead, the bodies were buried shallowly. The evidence lay in the careless nature of the grave goods. There was no clothing, there was only newspaper.

I do not accept this theory. I do not believe that the bodies had been buried in a rushed manner. Remember, in 1918 coffins were in short supply, with the pandemic raging; wooden coffins would have been even scarcer in the Arctic, where there are no real trees. In 1918, people buried their dead in whatever was available – including paper shrouds.

The second theory. I suggested that the bodies had perhaps been buried at a depth of 2.0 m and had been rising gradually over time. If the miners had been buried deep, the bodies might have been frozen for the first decades of their long rest, as opposed to having been exposed to alternate freezing and thawing for 80 years.

If the coffins had been rising over time, they would probably continue to do so after our reburying them and might ultimately resurface. My team's response: at least the project would provide answers regarding the presence of live virus. I remain concerned about how the families or the community might feel about resurfacing coffins containing Spanish influenza victims.

Prior to dinner, the team met to make sure that we were all communicating consistently. Members of Necropolis still strongly believed that there was a second row of coffins. Everyone voiced his or her opinion about whether the team should continue to dig further into the permafrost. Only Rod and I opposed further digging. The team would continue to dig.

After the important vote, I explained that I would be unable to pay my hotel bill, which would mount to over $5,000. I explained that I had the second-longest stay in Longyearbyen and therefore the second-most-expensive bill of all the team members. I explained that John Oxford had agreed to pay Alan's stay, the longest, and Tom's, the third longest. However, he would not cover my stay. I explained that I did not have the cash or credit and that I simply had no way to pay the amount. I had been raising this point since July. No one uttered a word.

After my request, Rob Webster unrolled a white T-shirt and passed it across the table to me: 'The T-shirt is for you.' On its front was a giant flu virus with the words 'Get a grippe' (another word for 'flu'). Rob had designed the shirt himself to distribute to participants at a meeting, and he asked me to wear it to our press conference the next day. Alan and Charles beamed, adding later, 'You have the respect of Rob Webster.' The neophyte had come a long way!

Dinner was a special treat that night, as Dr Christopher Longyear, grandson of J.M. Longyear, founder of Longyear City, had flown in to host a celebratory dinner. A generous gift! The night was even more special as Governor Olsen, Pastor Hoifodt, and school teacher Mork were all present. The governor entertained us with wonderful Arctic tales of romance and lost loves. And Charles and I thanked Longyear for his kindness.

Day 10. In the morning, the team began to dig below the seventh coffin. The ground was unstable (i.e., the water-sodden soil was subject to collapse). An entourage was dispatched to the governor's office to explain the risks involved in continuing the work. The governor made it clear that work should cease. She later visited the site to make sure that it did indeed stop.

The work at Longyearbyen was over. The precious samples had been collected, and Sir John Skehel left for home. As the team began moving the supplies downhill, Necropolis started backfilling the pit and restoring the site. The work would continue until there was no trace of our having been there and the restoration met with the approval of the governor of Svalbard.

We had a team meeting at eight p.m. John Oxford was livid. He demanded that we continue to dig. He raged that Roche, a funder of the project, was not happy about the outcome. After all, the project was, according to John, a disaster. He demanded that we come up with a scheme to dig or drill by morning. He would not accept that the work was over. We all explained that legally we had no right to continue. I said simply that there could be no digging, that I had promised that the work would be done safely. It was over.

He questioned, 'Couldn't we just go ahead? No one would know.'

'No, John. I would know.' Working was unsafe, and therefore we would not continue.

Charles and Alan then explained that legally and technically they could no longer work. Finally, Rob Webster raised his voice and explained that the governor would not allow us to dig.

John calmed down, but he still insisted that the project was a disaster. Rob then angrily expressed his disappointment regarding the exhumation. Disappointment? I had been there watching him do the work in the tent; there had been no disappointment. I had watched him stretch out his hand with anticipation for each important sample. He had looked awe-struck. Charles compared Rob's reaction with a child's response in a candy store. Moreover, had he forgotten his earlier speech about science? Science is about slow, methodical work. It is not about guessing. Rob, of all people, was guessing about the results.

I had got them to Longyearbyen, they had taken their samples, and some were still grumbling. I had waited six years to do the work. Couldn't they wait even a few months to undertake the analyses in the laboratory before they began declaring their disappointment? Even Rod, who was to test our samples at NIMR, was guessing that they were poor. He complained, 'The state of the material we've collected ... does not fill me with confidence.'[1] Rob apologized to me later for his outburst. He said that he was pleased by the amount of material and that our next job would be to wait for the results.

Day 11. At the morning press conference I explained that exploration of the permafrost was finished, because unusual climatic conditions had made work difficult and unsafe, and that the team believed strongly that the six graves examined were indeed those of the 1918 influenza victims. The stoppage was in keeping with the team's guiding principles – that the project have the highest safety standards. We then displayed Rob Webster's gift to me. Rob was pleased, and we all drew close.

Following the last press conference, Necropolis continued backfilling the pit and moving supplies downhill. An electrical supply was set up for shipping container no. 2, and the freezer, with its samples, was moved down from the tent into the container. Rod would now regularly check the freezer to make sure that it was functioning properly.

In the meantime, I still had no way of paying my hotel bill. Again, I approached John, who was no longer talking to me. He made it clear that my finances were not his worry. Roger, the head of Necropolis, a kindly gentleman, overhead the discussion. He privately informed me that Necropolis would cover my costs and would bill the team later. I was relieved. I could never thank him enough for his kindness.

Charles invited me to accompany him on a visit to SNSK's mine no. 3. I accepted gladly, as I wanted to learn what life was like for a miner. When we got on our tour bus to the mine, we learned that John and Esther Oxford would be accompanying us. As soon as we boarded the jitney, John turned to the other tourists and asked what they thought of the project. Esther was taping the responses. Charles and I were deeply embarrassed. John, though warned by Tom that it was illegal in Norway to record people covertly, continued to tape anyway.

The mine trip was fascinating. Dark, wind-blown tunnels led us deeper and deeper into the mountain. Old digging machinery lay abandoned in almost every recess. But I politely declined when we were given the opportunity to explore the two-foot crawl spaces.

Mining in the Arctic is very difficult even today. The mines are unusual, as the tunnels lie below the permafrost. The average temperature of the mines is –2.0°C to –4.0°C, but wind chill must be factored in, since a very strong wind blows through the dark, damp passages.

After we returned from our mining excursion, Esther Oxford interviewed Charles. He told me that he tried to avoid criticizing her father's actions. Esther admitted that her father had told her 'great amounts' of inside material. She asked Charles why he had banned her father from the tent. Charles turned off her recording microphone and explained that her father had some unusual characteristics that made him successful in his work, but that he did not want to discuss them with her. Esther persisted and turned on the microphone. Charles explained that he had lost all confidence in her father's ability to keep his word. Esther argued that her father was the only one who was brave enough to speak with the media. Charles told Esther that her father had broken the rules under which we were working and that either her father had to be stopped, or the governor would stop the project. Esther then 'asked questions which tried to lay blame.' She questioned my 'leadership and Alan's competence.' John was blaming Alan, who had planned and supervised the whole excavation so well, for the halting of work and the interpretation of the GPR results.

Day 12. Sunday was another rest day. I chose to sail to the Russian mining town of Pyramiden with Rod, Peter, and reporter Mary MacKenna.

The town would cease to exist by the end of the week, since the Russians were about to kill the main industry there. Months earlier, a community of 1,000 people had lived and worked there; on 30 August, only 80 remained. A forbidding sculpture of Lenin loomed above the abandoned sports centre and town, which was a mix of beautiful, old carved wooden Russian buildings and modern, concrete Soviet slabs. A greenhouse in which tomatoes and lettuce had once flourished and a barn that had once protected cattle and pigs stood forlorn and silent. We saw no one. It was as if everyone had stopped in mid-activity and fled before some unknown force.

After leaving Pyramiden, we sailed close to the tongue of a glacier protruding into the beautiful, sparkling, turquoise sea. The captain of our ship fished pieces of iceberg from the sea with a long hook in order to serve 'whisky on the bergs' to his passengers, who were so inclined. He explained that the glaciers of Svalbard were receding rapidly. My mind quickly raced ahead to concepts of global warming and questions of whether the miners' bodies would resurface. Bodies had floated to the surface of the ground throughout Svalbard. I wondered if the bodies of our miners would reappear.

Generally, the team did not accept the concept of global warming. The world's governing body on global warming, the Intergovernmental Panel on Climate Change (IPCC), a joint venture of the United Nations Environmental Programme and the World Meteorological Organization, however, suggests that Earth will get warmer over the next century.[4, 5]

I thought of the conflict among scientists regarding global warming. All scientists agree that Earth has a natural greenhouse effect, which maintains its mean temperature of about 15°C. The greenhouse effect is necessary and good. Without it, the planet's mean temperature would be about 33°C colder than at present, and no water would exist in liquid form.[6-7] Greenhouse gases, such as water vapour, carbon dioxide (CO_2), and methane, allow the sun's short-wave, or ultra-violet, radiation to pass through the atmosphere to Earth. Earth in turn gives off long-wave, or infrared, radiation, which warms the planet when trapped by greenhouse gases.[7]

Scientists agree that humans are adding greenhouse gases to the atmosphere. The evidence speaks for itself. Over the past two million years, atmospheric levels of CO_2 have ranged between 200 and 280 parts per million (ppm). About the time of the industrial revolution, concentrations suddenly began to escalate. CO_2, when first monitored in 1958 at Mauna Loa, Hawaii, measured 315 ppm. By 1988, it measured 350 ppm; and by 1994, 358 ppm.[5] Scientists agree that as concentrations continue to rise, they enhance the greenhouse effect.[8]

Scientists disagree, however, on the amount of warming and the rate of temperature change.[7] The IPCC predicts that atmospheric CO_2 will double, if not triple, over pre-industrial levels by 2100. Models project globally averaged surface temperature to warm 1.4–5.8°C by 2100 relative to 1990.[9–10] Such a change may not seem significant. But a temperature decrease of 2.0–4.0°C is enough to bring on a near-hemispheric ice age. Moreover warming at the Poles will be much greater than for Earth as a whole. For example, northern Canada's winter mean temperature is expected to increase by a shocking 8.0–10.0°C.[11] Warming will profoundly affect Earth, causing sea levels to rise and glaciers and permafrost to melt.[4] Should the thermal regime of the permafrost in Longyearbyen be altered, the miners' bodies could float to the surface of the cemetery.

The team had consulted outside specialists (1997) on the best way to rebury the miners to prevent future jacking of the bodies or frost heave. Necropolis followed the consultants' suggestions, and the governor's office was to monitor the site for any changes following reburial. If there was any deterioration, the team was prepared to do further restoration, with money so dedicated.

We took every precaution to prevent the bodies from resurfacing. Nevertheless, they may float to the surface in the future. In other parts of the world, bodies in permafrost may also rise, not because of disturbance, but because of warming.

Tom returned to Longyearbyen, and John Oxford and Rob Webster left for their respective homes. Necropolis completed backfilling the burial pit and kept moving all supplies downhill. They also began dismantling the soil-storage tank and removing the ground protection.

While Necropolis toiled, Rod packed our tissue samples into steel shipping drums and continued his checks on the freezer. At the same time, Tom and Alan arranged a meeting at UNIS to discuss the project with the community the day after my departure. They would tell the community the final result of the expedition.

Day 14. I was going home. Prior to my departure, Tom said that I had done a good job. Rob had given me a T-shirt. And Rod volunteered, 'I guess I should thank you. I guess none of us would ever have been here if it wasn't for you.'

Tom then warned me that if I had thought the expedition was a struggle, authorship on the future paper discussing results would produce an even greater fight. He cautioned that I could trust no one. He told me nothing I hadn't appreciated for a long time. I had fought so hard to get a lab agreement to avoid such a conflict.

Tom and I also agreed that I would have a difficult time obtaining updates on the testing of samples and getting the samples out of Britain for shipment to Norway and Canada. Sir John's NIMR, which had first isolated influenza in 1933, wanted to be the first to isolate the 1918 virus.

Following our talk, I boarded my plane for home. It would be a pleasant flight with Charles, Barry, and Peter. My thoughts: the work had proceeded safely. We had the samples. I should have been exhilarated; instead, I was exhausted – exhausted because team relations had been so very difficult. We were a team. Team members should treat one another with trust and respect. Our members often showed little of either. However, whenever I had thought that I couldn't take even one more minute, Peter, Alan, or Charles had buoyed my spirits with an encouraging word.

In the first days of September, according to Alan's detailed log, Necropolis relaid the turf in the cemetery and removed the turf-storage platform. The crew disconnected the soil-storage tank. It dismantled the site protection and moved the tent and all supplies downhill. Necropolis replaced the curb stones surrounding the graves. It hauled the head stones and crosses uphill and re-erected them. And it removed all remaining waste from the site. Photographs of the site following the clean-up still amaze me. Necropolis, professional and caring to the utmost degree, had done a remarkable job.

While the clean-up continued, Rod conducted the all-important checks on the freezer. And on 3 September, the first case of tissue samples left for London. Back at the cemetery, Pastor Hoifodt blessed the work site, and Tom laid the wreath purchased weeks earlier.

Alan replaced the original fence around the cemetery on 5 September. He also arranged for a plaque to be erected by the governor's office. The inscription reads: 'The 1918 Spanish flu Influenza Research Project. This site was excavated in August, 1998, as part of a medical archaeology research project to study the 1918 Spanish influenza virus. Please do not walk on the grave plot, as the ground and the vegetation are not yet fully stabilized.'

Necropolis began packing the shipping containers and disconnecting the electrical feed to the work area. Tom departed for Oslo. Regular checks continued on the freezer until 6 September, when the second case of samples was shipped.

On 7 September the waste container was removed, while the men continued packing the shipping containers. Rod finally left for London. Packing of the shipping containers, however, lasted into the next day, during which Alan did a final site survey to clear litter, before departing for home.

The containers were transported to the dock by truck on 9 September. Necropolis repeated the litter pick-up and departed the next day. 'And then there were none.'

Part Five

Decoding the Virus

16 Waiting for Results

November 1998–October 1999

When I returned home, I did no work on the project for a while. I knew that Rod Daniels, who would test our samples (Phase III) required time to catch up on missed work. And as it turned out, the staff at NIMR's BSL 4 laboratory needed an additional two months to become operational and ready to begin testing the samples. We had flown the precious material on two separate flights to London in case a plane was lost, in containers that had multi-layer, mechanical, and thermal protection. The lab at Mill Hill was to have been functional in August. Sir John Skehel had convinced the team to send the samples to his laboratory with the promise that it would be operational in time – unlike the Canadian facility.

During the hiatus, the world's media repeatedly requested results. I explained that the samples had yet to be analysed, since the BSL 4 lab had still to open. Journalists and scientists alike speculated continually about the nature of the samples. For example, Dr Jeffrey Taubenberger, who was not present in Longyearbyen and was no longer a team member, thought our chances of recovering (viral) RNA from the bodies 'very close to zero.' 'The Longyearbyen burial site ... could be very acidic. If that's the case, the acidic environment does a great job of chewing up RNA. Freezing and thawing would help that process as well.'[1]

In November, I heard from Governor Olsen: 'It's been a pleasure for me and my entire staff to get to know you and to learn of your effective and well organized international project. We are pleased concerning the cleanup and restoration of the site. I've not heard any complaints whatsoever.' This would be her last official letter to me, as she was finishing her post and leaving Longyearbyen. The new governor would continue to monitor the site for the team. A year after the expedition, the new governor reported to Tom Bergan, 'The site was inspected on August 1 and September 21 (1999). Everything is ok and further need for ... refill/removal of ground mass is not necessary at this time.' Tom reported to the team: 'On both occasions the site looked as if we had not been there.'

On 16 November, I was able to write to the team's SAG, 'It is with great delight that I inform you that the BSL4 Lab in Mill Hill will likely be operational this week. This means that it will be possible to begin testing the samples.'

Testing the Samples, November 1998–May 1999

My fax continued, 'It is important that we all remember how the samples were to be tested. It was agreed in Longyearbyen that the samples would be tested for safety (i.e. the samples would be tested for the presence of live virus) at Mill Hill. Once the samples were deemed safe, they would then be shipped to labs in the United States, Canada and Norway. This would give the four countries equal access to the samples. PCR testing [i.e., genetic decoding of the virus] 'was not to take place at Mill Hill until after the samples were deemed safe.'

Despite the team's agreement in Longyearbyen and my fax, John Oxford and Sir John Skehel faxed me that PCR testing should take place at the same time as testing for live virus – or, in Sir John's words, 'GO IN PARALLEL.' Initially, the plan had been for the samples to be tested 'IN PARALLEL' at the different labs, with the team and all labs confirming the results before releasing them to the scientific community. I feared that NIMR would get results ahead of the other labs and publish them first, to its benefit and everyone else's detriment.

On 17 November, Alan Heginbottom wrote to Sir John: 'Testing for infectivity is to be done at Mill Hill. If the samples are not infectious, representative suites of medical samples should be shipped to designated labs in Canada and USA for PCR and virological analysis, and to Norway for bacteriological analysis. All the non-medical samples should be shipped to Norway for conservation and evaluation by museums and archives people ... Once samples have been shipped to the labs in Canada, Norway and USA, then PCR and virological analysis should commence.' Following the round of faxes, there was silence from Mill Hill.

In the meantime Esther Oxford's article appeared in print. On 18 November, Tom Bergan faxed me regarding Esther's piece, which 'quite clearly scandalizes you. It also talks in a downgrading manner about how we had a microbiologist trying [*sic*] to lecture us on virology.' In Britain, virology is a distinct discipline, whereas in Norway, it is merely a subdiscipline of microbiology. Tom continued, 'In contrast, the pillars of the project, Professor John Oxford and Mrs. Gillian Oxford, are projected in rather flattering terms.' Roger Webber also from Necropolis enclosed Esther Oxford's 'rather controversial article.'

While awaiting news from Britain, I requested the project's financial report – a complete breakdown of finances, especially outstanding invoices. I also needed to know that Peter Lewin had been fully reimbursed for his Norway trip. I wrote to John, 'As you know, he is a valued member of the team; both his contribution in the tent and his medical expertise were most valuable. It is imperative that this project and our respective Institutions are not perceived as leaving a trail of unpaid invoices.' Finally, 'I understand ... that you are no longer paying my administrative costs. I understand that these were passed on to St. Jude ... As you know, the [NIH] grant does not cover my administrative costs. It was agreed (at the Workshop at NIMR) that our Roche grant would cover my administrative costs. There has been no change in this policy. I will, therefore, re-send my invoices and expect full payment.'

John Oxford responded on 22 December. 'We cannot guarantee to pay expenses after the exhumation so I am afraid you will have to direct them to your University. I am sure they will be understanding.' John was denying me reimbursement from our joint research grant. On 28 January 1999, he continued, 'We are still sorting out the Svalbard Hotel, etc. I am still receiving some claims from team members where there was clear agreement about expenses. I am sure that you remember that Peter Lewin was in a gray area where there was no guarantee of payment.' We had agreed at the University of Toronto meeting (15 April 1998) that all team members would go to Longyearbyen. Shortly thereafter, John decided on his own that there would be no money for Peter. I called John and followed up my phone call with a fax explaining that all team members were to go to Longyearbyen; I also asked John to put it in writing that Peter would go to Svalbard and that his expenses would be paid in full. John provided written assent.

John had clearly changed his mind in January 1999. I called him and followed up with a fax. 'There was no gray area. I have verbal and written communication from you that Peter would be paid. There is no ranking of team members. You have wrongly ranked human beings in order of your preference.'

There was silence from NIMR until January 1999, when Rod Daniels explained to me that no live virus had yet been detected in the samples. This was not surprising. The expert panel on influenza at NIH had estimated the risk of finding live virus to be 10^{-18} if the bodies were found in the true permafrost. The probability was greatly reduced when the bodies were found in the active layer of the permafrost.

PCR was proceeding in conjunction with testing for live virus – despite the team's Longyearbyen agreement. Perhaps NIMR would respect Robert Webster, who had first invited Sir John to the project. I called Rob, who was in Hong Kong. His assistant suggested that I fax her my concerns, which she would then fax to Rob.

I wrote on 27 January, '**URGENT! Could you please get this fax to Dr. Webster ASAP?** ... I received an update from Rod Daniels. I am sure that you have also received the update.' I explained that Rod proposed to proceed with PCR screening of samples in conjunction with looking for live virus. 'Tom has spoken with Rod and is pleased. Norway will get their samples after isolation (of live virus) has been attempted because Norway does not have a BSL 4 lab; Norway will undertake bacteriological studies. I am **very** concerned about you (Rob). When do you want your samples? I thought that you wanted to do PCR. Please let me know your wants ASAP ... The Canadian lab is still interested in receiving specimens for testing. They, too, would like to do PCR as was agreed. USAMRIID has agreed to hold the Canadian samples until the Canadian lab is ready. I must proceed in making this happen. I am willing to make this happen for you too.'

There was no response from Rob to my fax. I called Rob's assistant and was asked to fax the letter of 27 January again. To ensure delivery, his aide would mail the correspondence in her next shipping to Rob. Again, no response. I would repeat the exercise one more time.

While waiting for a response from Rob, I faxed Rod Daniels to inquire if there were any PCR results and to learn how the Canadian samples might be shipped. I received no response. But correspondence from Alan to Rod prompted Sir John to write, 'I read your E-mail to Rod about progress with analyzing the samples and plans for further analysis and *thought it was time to involve the SAG* [emphasis added]. ... Both infectivity tests ... and PCR screening for influenza RNA are proceeding in parallel; the latter (PCR) is quicker and will, therefore, be completed sooner ... Plans for additional analysis elsewhere are of two sorts: (a) further analysis of samples that we have screened and shown to be negative (for live virus) will be available for work in lower containment laboratories straight away. We will need to know the addresses ... (b) analysis of samples that we have not screened or plan not to screen are available for work in containment IV laboratories immediately, as in fact, they always have been.'

Sir John's laboratory had broken our agreement. NIMR was testing for infectivity and PCR screening at the same time. NIMR could choose the best samples for itself and share its discards. Our British colleagues appeared to be competing with the rest of us.

In April, Tom joined me in asking the whereabouts of Norway's samples and the results of the analyses. He faxed me on 10 April, 'Heard from London about the samples? We have not seen even a trace of the promised samples here in Oslo.' On 21 May he asked of NIMR, 'Please let me know how the study is progressing. Please let us have our samples A.S.A.P.'

Also in April, Dr Harvey Artsob of Health Canada began asking when Canada would obtain its samples. On the 19th, he wrote Sir John: 'The purpose of this letter is to seek confirmation from you that tissue specimens are available for my laboratory and, if so, to inquire as to what specific types of tissue were collected for analysis.'

While waiting for any PCR results, I received a call from Gina Kolata, medical reporter from the *New York Times*, who wanted to interview me for her book. I ignored her request, but she was not about to give up. She sent more faxes, voice-mail messages, and e-mails. Eventually, she caught me at the University of Windsor. She asked if I had received her request and if I would be willing to be interviewed. I was brutally honest. 'I do not feel comfortable speaking with you, as you have been dishonest with me in the past.' She suggested that if I would submit to an interview, she would allow me to see the last version of her chapter concerning my work for my approval.

That seemed fair. I agreed to be interviewed – not only because of her offer, but because I was concerned that John Oxford might speak for me and give his version of the project, as he had done with his daughter. Gina's chapter arrived by e-mail shortly after our conversation. Later, she called me and asked what I thought. I said, 'There are numerous errors and there are outright lies.' I said that the term 'Svalberg' (referring to Svalbard) appeared repeatedly. She said that she knew that I 'would feel awful about it [the chapter]' and that she was 'sorry.' But she was only 'writing what others were saying.' I understood that she could not change their stories, but she could certainly fix errors in my story. We set up a time to do the corrections, and I arranged that my parents be in the room for the phone call as witnesses. I no longer did anything without the presence of a witness or a lawyer. I spent well over an hour with her on the phone. She had attributed phrases to me that I had never uttered. I said, 'Then be fair, and take them out.'

I asked her why she was leaving out pertinent information. She had written, 'Should Duncan go ahead with her project that might unleash live flu virus, one of the most deadly viruses ever known, when he [Taubenberger] could get the same information with utter safety.' I asked her why she did not mention that the team had grappled with the same question. 'Dr Taubenberger,' I repeated, 'had been invited to a meeting at the Centers for Disease Control to present his work, and we decided to go forward with the project because more information was needed.' Moreover, he had agreed to join our project. Clearly, he also felt that more information was needed.

I asked Gina why she did not ask if Hultin's work 'might unleash live flu virus, one of the most deadly viruses ever known,' especially when his expedition had been planned in just one week and no safety protocols had been taken? Our expedition, in contrast, had been planned over six years, with two years spent on developing safety protocols. She agreed to remove the sentences in question.

There was another draft. New quotes from John Oxford included a fabrication of his wanting Taubenberger to be part of the Spitsbergen project. My lawyer told me to put Kolata 'on notice'; if she used John's material, I could sue her. At the time of our discussion, she stated that I had seen the final draft of the chapter. Legally, if the editor wanted to make any small changes, minor modifications were permitted. From prior experience, however, I knew that there were likely to be major changes.

In November 1999, reporter Maryn McKenna of the *Atlanta Journal Constitution* called and warned me against reading the book. Gina had 'gotten hold of Esther Oxford's article and inserted Esther's comments throughout her chapter (the "final" chapter which I had approved).' I told Maryn that Gina had told me that she couldn't 'find anything to fault [me] on.' I had 'done such good work'; she commented on 'the time spent on the safety,' and added, 'You really put together a remark-able project." Maryn informed me that Gina had used Esther's deroga-tory comments regarding my personality, my appearance, and my dress. (Some people, however, thought that we had done good work. I was invited to present the annual Arnold G. Wedum Memorial Lecture to the annual conference of the American Biological Safety Association, 17–20 October 1999 in St Louis, Missouri. I was awarded this lecture-ship and a plaque 'in recognition of outstanding work that provided greater knowledge in the field of biosafety.' Our team's safety proto-cols had been recognized by academics, government officials, and experts in biological safety.)

Results, May–October 1999

In May 1999 I received the most tremendous fax from Alan: 'I spoke with Rod in mid-March, who told me that he was getting interesting results.' I read the fax over and over. I then phoned Alan. 'Alan, I just got your fax. I'm in shock. We're getting results. I can't believe it. After all the difficulty, after the press's deriding the project, after John's com-plaining that the expedition was a bust, and after all the unpleasant-ness, we're getting results. I'm over the moon.'

Then I asked, 'How did you find out?' I explained that both Tom and I had been asking for months. Alan had 'caught Rod by surprise,' he had 'caught him off guard.' I left Rod another voice-mail message explaining that I knew that we had results. An e-mail from Rod fol-lowed. 'We have screened small pieces of all the soft tissue samples (30 in total) from all 6 bodies (most from number 1) for virus isolation in Primary Monkey Kidney cells (PMK) ... On the PCR front, I have concentrated on HA as this is the gene for which we have the largest range of primers and have a number of observations. a) Fragment sizes generated are 100-150 base pairs. b) Have got signal from brain, lung, liver, and kidney (this is new compared to what Taubenberger has). c) The sequence we have (~800 base pairs in total) is not identical to Taubenberger but we are still missing the more informative regions of the gene (primers are designed and on order).' More work was to fol-low: 'to look at bone marrow and tooth pulp for isolation and PCR ... Without going into detail this is where we are.' Rod reported: '... media interest has diminished in the last few months and I have been left alone to get on with the work quietly (much as Taubenberger has done) – there is also the very real problem that if too much is "leaked" to the media, from whatever source, that it could prevent us from publishing in prestigious journals. To limit the possibility of the latter, the fewer people who know precisely where we are the better.' He added: 'If only the Svalbard samples had been as good as we all had hoped for, the analyses would be much further advanced.'

I called Alan – I wanted more information, recent details. I knew that Rod would ignore any further voice mail messages. Alan suggested that I try calling Rod at home.

Rod was clearly agitated by my call. 'I can't talk to you, Kirsty.' Why couldn't he talk to me? 'I could get into trouble.' Trouble from whom? 'Sir John doesn't want me talking.'

'Rod, it's my project. I started it. The team did it together. We have an agreement.'

'Kirsty, I'm not part of the SAG. Don't put me in the middle. There's a lot riding on this. People' s reputations are at stake.'

'Rod, I understand that. Some of you have derided the project, some of you have derided me, and now that you're getting results from the team's samples you won't share the exciting finds. It is dishonest. My reputation is at stake, too.'

'No, people who have invested their careers in flu research: people like Sir John and Rob Webster.'

'Rod, that's insulting.'

'I'm sorry.'

'What about Tom? Has Tom been told? You mention that the virologists know.'

'Tom doesn't know. He likes the media too much. He'll give away the results.'

'Rod, it is outrageous that Tom and the whole SAG have not been informed. Tom arranged everything on the Norwegian side. And Norway gave us the right to obtain those samples. Please tell Tom. I will trust that you will do so.'

'Fine.'

'Look Rod, I don't want you in the middle. How do you want me to handle this? Should I write to Sir John.'

'Yes. Kirsty, I have to go.' The phone clicked. The line went dead.

I wrote to Sir John on 24 May and copied the correspondence to the SAG. 'I am writing to you in order to: (1) establish an appropriate reporting mechanism regarding the Svalbard samples; and (2) make sure that the countries involved in the project will be receiving their samples as agreed in Longyearbyen. The NIMR was entrusted by the

SAG to search for live virus and then distribute the samples. Your lab is currently performing the analyses and is housing the samples. We require distribution. I understand from Rod that good progress is being made; this is very exciting. I was dismayed to learn, however, that the "influenza people" on the team already had an outline of the data. It is disappointing that I must remind the "influenza people" that this project is run by the project leader and the SAG. It is important to recognize the contribution of all scientists who contributed to this multidisciplinary project.'

We were now in Phase III – the laboratory analysis. 'Phase III will be run in the same fashion (that is, with complete information sharing) as Phases I and II.' I asked Sir John to 'update me at regular fixed intervals – as frequently as every three weeks ... I no longer want to have to beg for updates on the project that I founded. And I do not want Rod to be put in an uncomfortable or compromising position.' After receiving updates, I would then 'pass on the necessary information to the SAG.'

I wrote to Rod Daniels on 23 June to 'request an update regarding the testing of the Svalbard samples, as previously requested in my letter of May 24th, 1999 to Sir John Skehel. I would appreciate a detailed synopsis of what tests have been run on what samples. I would appreciate the synopsis as soon as possible, as the update was requested for June 18th, 1999.'

Sir John responded on 24 June and copied his fax to the SAG. 'To avoid any further communications until there is something actually to report I should say that since the samples arrived in our Cat 1V from Longyearbyen, primarily Rod Daniels and his Co-worker ... have made extensive attempts to isolate virus in numerous tissue culture cells, as yet to no avail in terms of identifying an influenza virus. *To expedite further analyses* of the samples so that they may make them available for use outside Cat IV by other members of the 1918 influenza team, *they have also done PCR on the same samples*. This work is still in progress and there are no data to currently report' (emphasis added). His laboratory appeared to be trying to help, but his people were doing the work before any other country could even look at the samples.

I responded on the 30th. 'I understand that you wanted "to avoid further communications." Unfortunately, your letter leaves me requiring further communication. You stated that there are no data currently to report. An E-mail message from Rod (in May) clearly states that there are "observations," which are briefly described. The "observations" were further confirmed in a follow-up phone call to Rod. 'As a result of the E-mail message and phone call, I wrote to you on May 24th, 1999, asking to be updated at regular fixed intervals. I am now informed that there are no data to currently report. This is especially confusing, as I have learned that researchers in the States know what tests have been performed and what the results have been.' (I learned the latter from Canadian scientists who wished to remain anonymous.) 'Please send me a report detailing: (1) the complete catalogue of samples; (2) what samples have been tested; and (3) and what results have been obtained from what samples. I will then pass the information on to the SAG.'

Tom wrote to Sir John on 2 July requesting Norway's samples and results. 'I still have not been able to give any other information to our Ministry than that your laboratory is neither answering questions nor shipping back the specimens as was foreseen.'

Sir John responded on the same day. 'I don't quite understand your fax of July 2nd – I did not receive a letter from you about sending any of the samples to Norway. We are still in the progress of testing for infectious virus in Containment IV and until these tests are completed to the satisfaction of the virologists, none of the samples will be sent to less than Containment IV labs. That has always been the situation and until the tests are complete that's how it will remain. The status report is as I wrote to Kirsty and until it changes I will not be writing her or any other member of the SAG.' Tom added to Sir John's response, 'The enclosed is very sad. That arrogance!'

On 5 July Tom wrote back to Sir John. 'Your wording in your fax ... is rather terse. I chaired a session on influenza last week at the International Congress of Chemotherapy. Rob Webster was among the speakers. I had the pleasure of talking also with John Oxford; he told me about some of the findings, i.e. that an enterovirus [a virus that enters the body through the gastrointestinal tract and multiplies there] has been found. Rob Webster had no further information. It would be most appropriate if you could give me an interim status report. The Ministry finds it appropriate to be updated, as a year has soon passed since the project started actively in Longyearbyen.

Sir John responded to Tom on 22 July: 'To my knowledge no viruses whatsoever have been recovered from any of the samples that were taken in Spitsbergen. I don't know where John Oxford got his information but it's news to me, and I suspect completely incorrect. I assure you that whenever there is anything to tell the SAG I will do so with pleasure.'

On 11 August, I contacted Rod regarding shipment of samples to the Canadian laboratory. I wrote, 'Dr. Artsob first wrote Sir John Skehel on April 19th, 1999. Sir John agreed that samples would be available to the Canadian lab and suggested that Dr. Artsob contact you directly. Dr. Artsob E-mailed you on July 7th, 1999. He is concerned that he has not had a reply.'

I updated my team on 9 September. 'Unfortunately, I have had great difficulty learning of the progress myself. However, I will share with you what I have been able to glean from our esteemed British colleagues ... It appears that we have "observations" regarding the samples. This is exciting. It is important, however, that we publish the "observations" in scientific journals. Therefore I will remind you that we all agreed not to communicate with the media regarding the analyses and results at our final team meeting in Longyearbyen. It also appears that there is some hesitation to correspond with the Canadian lab.'

In the meantime, unbeknown to me, John Oxford had invited some members of the team to a conference that he was organizing with the 'backing of Sir John Skehel and Robert Webster.' 'Influenza – Past, Present and Future: Genetics of Virulence and Pathogenicity' was to take place 15–16 November 1999 in London.

When Charles received my fax of 9 September indicating results, he was not surprised.

'No, I figured we had results when I received John's invitation to his conference. Are you going to it?'

'What conference? What are you talking about, Charles?'

'John is holding a conference in November. Rod is going to speak about reverse genetics to reconstruct the 1918 virus.'

'What? He's going to release our results.'

'It looks that way, Kirsty. You've got to go.'

I immediately phoned Tom. 'Tom, John Oxford is hosting a conference on influenza and Rod is going to speak about reconstructing the 1918 virus. Were you invited?'

'No.'

'Neither was I.'

'I don't think John likes us very much. '

'Was Bjorn Berdal invited? Tom, I'm going to ask John for my invitation to his meeting. I'll fax you a copy of the invitation, which Charles is currently faxing to me.'

On 20 September, I faxed John Oxford. 'I am writing to you in order to let you know that my invitation to your conference has yet to arrive. However, I will be delighted to attend. I will also be delighted to speak. I would like to speak before Dr. Daniel's presentation. I trust that you will accommodate me – and at no cost, as I am the project leader. I trust that the whole team has been invited.' I expressed surprise at Taubenberger's being invited, given John Oxford's earlier attitude towards him. On the 21st, I wrote, 'I am still waiting for my invitation.'

John responded the next day. 'I think you have been misinformed about the Influenza Conference in London. This is a scientific meeting about the genetics of virulence and not about Spitsbergen ... There are no expenses available and no opportunities for a speaker's spot ... Dr. Reid and Dr. Taubenberger's contribution should be most interesting because they have now sequenced 3 genes of the 1918 virus ... I expect if we all reconstruct the events of the USA/Canadian/Norway/UK project we would remember differently, and I have no doubt that we all, you included, did things which seemed for the best at the time.'

I responded on the 23rd. 'I was not "misinformed" about your meeting. I was not "informed" – i.e. I was not invited. However, I will be attending. You did invite Dr. Charles Smith (pathologist) and Mr. Alan Heginbottom (geologist) from the Spitsbergen expedition. Clearly, their specific fields are not related to the "genetics of virulence." And clearly, you are inviting participants from the Spitsbergen expedition.' I indicated my disappointment that Tom Bergan, Bjorn Berdal, and I had not been invited. 'It is of concern that Dr. Daniels will be speaking about "Use of reverse transcriptase genetics to reconstruct the 1918 virus." Information regarding the 1918 virus originates from two sources: Dr. Taubenberger's samples; and the Spitsbergen samples. You have invited Dr. Taubenberger to speak. I must again ask you to allow me to speak about Spitsbergen. It is imperative to put the Spitsbergen samples in their correct context. I do not "reconstruct" events. I have minutes of all the meetings. I have every correspondence. I also have corroboration of events, which you suggest that I remember differently from yourself.'

While I was communicating with John Oxford, Tom was asking Sir John about samples and results. On 16 September, he wrote that he had to 'make a report to the Norw. Ministry of Health now that a year has passed. I am a bit perturbed that we have no information nor any specimens returned to Norway.' He enclosed a strong report to the ministry and advised Sir John that he would send his report in two weeks. On the 21st, he gave Sir John another chance. 'I would not be surprised if you find the enclosed rather terse, but this is the way it appears to us and any positive information will mellow our feeling. I have not sent the previous version to the government, but have kept the date on my letter as Oct. 1, 1999, since I have to respond.'

Sir John responded the same day. 'I would be extremely disappointed if you send the letter that you copied to me today to anyone. It is simply not true that I refused to answer questions about the status of the laboratory work. I refer you especially to my fax to you dated 22 July [explaining that no virus had been found and 'that whenever there is anything to tell the SAG I will do so with pleasure'], my fax to Kirsty Duncan, copied to you ... I am sure that in light of these communications your statement in the last sentence would not be acceptable to me.' As for material, 'we cannot send samples back to you until they have been tested for virus under Containment IV conditions. This is taking a long time and if you can obtain a laboratory with Containment IV facilities you will be welcome to receive any samples that you require.' Finally, 'Please let me know if you are still unsure about the status of the samples or of progress in their analyses.'

On 1 October, Tom drafted another letter to Norway's Ministry of Health. 'Regrettably we have not received any specimens back and the Director, Sir John Skehel, has refused to answer questions about the status of the laboratory work, except to say that no enterovirus has been isolated.'

On the 7th, Tom gave up communicating with John Skehel and wrote to John Oxford. 'John Skehel refuses to release our specimens, which is ridiculous now that repeated attempts to isolate live virus have failed and everyone is convinced that there could not be any live virus after such a long time and those storage conditions anyway. Consequently, my annual report to the Norwegian authorities will not be good ... He has been given a chance to improve two drafts of an annual report, without rendering constructive input. We very much regret being kept in the total dark. His attitude is imperial, unacceptable, inconsistent with expected scientific openness among collaborators, would appear to contradict the spirit of the permissions given, and the MOU, and will be surprising to the Norwegian authorities. I would appreciate if you could do something about this. Although now overdue, I will stall until next Monday before sending the official.' Tom's report would be in the public domain and when picked up by journalists would most likely be scandalous.

I received a rather pleasant fax from John Oxford. I thanked him for his correspondence and wrote, 'It was pleasing to hear that you "would like to work more nicely again." Unfortunately, some of your comments in the press do not represent this collegial attitude. I have learned some disappointing things from our colleagues ... However, I look forward to this new working relationship.'

And on the 8th, Tom wrote one more fax to John Skehel. 'You have not responded constructively, but with unacceptable negative bursts and flak. This has had an imperial air about it, as if you consider other members of the SAG as subordinates. I react to this attitude most strongly ... Enclosed please find a third draft. If you want that changed, for the third time, please tell me how you would like the wording to be, and save your less elegant terms to the effect that you strongly object without supplementing with constructive criticism.'

Four days later, Rod Daniels finally faxed Tom a copy of his May e-mail discussing the results. The Canadian laboratory received the e-mail a month earlier, on 27 September, with a catalogue of all the samples. Tom had forced NIMR to share the results. And on 25 October, Tom wrote a positive letter to the Norwegian ministry. Two days later, John Oxford reimbursed Peter Lewin, Hospital for Sick Children, for the expedition thirteen months earlier.

A year after Longyearbyen, my team had results – unpublished. The next step would be to publish the findings. No doubt, a new battle would develop regarding authorship and credit. Perhaps the first winds of the storm were already stirring with John Oxford's conference, scheduled for mid-November. I needed to be present for the discussions regarding reconstruction of the 1918 virus. I had to protect Norway's interests, and the team's.

17 Fighting for Norway, Fighting for Canada

11–16 November 1999

After John Oxford informed me that there was no room for a speaker's spot at 'Influenza – Past, Present and Future,' I tried to obtain travel money for the conference on 15–16 November 1999. I had now spent over $70,000; John Oxford had decided (22 December 1998) that he was no longer paying my administrative costs from our joint Roche grant. By early November 1999, I still had no funding and had to give up hope of attending the conference.

Phone Alert

On Thursday, 11 November, I received several calls from the British media. One gentleman asked me if I was part of 'John Oxford's Spitsbergen expedition.' I explained that I was the project leader and that John was a member of my project. Could I expand on his information about the team's results, which were to be released at a press conference on Tuesday, 16 November, in London? John Oxford – with the backing of Rob Webster and Sir John Skehel – was going to release the results, not only to the scientific community, but also to the world. I remembered John Oxford's disappointment regarding the samples and Rob Webster's words, 'None of us want to take what you've achieved.' I also recalled Rod Daniel's saying: 'There is also the very real problem that if too much is "leaked" to the media, from whatever source, that it could prevent us from publishing in prestigious journals.'

I asked what results the reporter had. He gave me new information – information that I had been requesting since May. I asked from whom he had obtained it. He had spoken with Oxford but refused to tell me who had given him the results. The source seemed abundantly clear. I explained that, if he could not be honest with me, I couldn't speak with him and the conversation was over.

I immediately called Charles, who had been thinking for months of attending the conference. I told him what had transpired and added, 'I guess I'll have to go. I don't know where I'll get the money.' My parents were adamant that they would cover the cost, as their 'contribution to the project.'

I asked Charles, who had been invited but not funded, if he could join me. 'Charles, I know that it is a huge request, a huge financial commitment.' He said that that didn't bother him; he knew I needed the support. Unfortunately, the trip was impossible because of his work commitments. He asked what I would do if the conference organizers wouldn't admit me. I said that I didn't think that they would be that stupid. I had to do what I thought was right. I had to thank Norway publicly and get credit for my shunned team members – whatever the backlash.

Early Friday morning, I called Leslie Papp at the *Toronto Star*. He had initially covered the story but was no longer on the medical beat. He passed me over to Tanya Talaga, who arrived shortly after noon at my house. We began going over the history of the project and the key faxes. I had not been invited to the London conference, and John Oxford had informed me that the conference was not about Spitsbergen.

During the meeting, my husband, Robert, called. He rightly assumed that John Oxford would have a public relations company for the conference. John's Retroscreen Virology Company gave Robert the number for OCC – the PR company for the event. Roche was backing the conference and no longer using Hill & Knowlton. Robert then called OCC and asked for the press release. As Robert and I spoke on the one telephone, he faxed me the British release on a second phone line in the house. Robert's last words: 'Don't panic. We'll make it right.'

Media Alert

I walked to my bedroom. I read the release as it rolled out of the fax machine. There in the middle of it were the words: 'The symposium will provide the first opportunity to hear the data from the Spitsbergen expedition undertaken by Professor Oxford and his team.'

I then walked to the living-room, where Tanya was waiting. I was shaking; I could barely hold the paper. All I could say is, 'He's stealing. He's stealing from Norway, and he's stealing from the team. It's academic piracy.'

It was theft from Norway. The samples had not been returned to Norway, and the country had not been informed of the results. Without Norway's permission to undertake the work, there would have been no new findings, nothing for John Oxford to announce. From the media alert, I understood why the British journalist had asked if I was part of Oxford's expedition. I had to fly to England to ensure proper credit for Norway, for key Norwegian team members, and for Canadian members omitted from the invitation list. While Tanya waited to continue the interview, I booked tickets to London for Robert and me. We would leave the next day, Saturday, and arrive Sunday morning, the day before the conference.

Tanya was most understanding of the interruptions. She was extremely diligent. She explained that she would have to talk to the others involved before writing any story. I obtained permission from Charles, Peter, Alan, and Tom before releasing their phone numbers to her. She said that she would need to speak with Oxford. I did not want to ask his permission, as I did not want to have to speak to him, and it might alert him to the fact that I was coming – although I had previously informed him that I would be present, I had never actually registered for the meeting. She would have to chase down his numbers herself.

Before Robert and I left for London, my Canadian colleagues all talked with Tanya a number of times. During my last conversation with Tanya, I promised to call her as soon as we had any further news of the conference.

Sunday afternoon, we called my parents from a red telephone booth near Hyde Park in London. My mother answered the phone and said, 'Tanya's article is out and it's excellent. It couldn't be better!' She read snippets to me in which Alan said, 'Kirsty was getting screwed by these guys and it is really too bad, because she put a lot of blood, sweat and tears into this project,' and Peter said, 'an agreement was made that, before any publication or announcement was made by any of our group, that we should all consult together. And that obviously hasn't happened for whatever reason. '

'Kirsty,' Mom cautioned, 'you have the fight of your life ahead of you tomorrow.'

Conference: Day One

We arrived early at the conference on 15 November and surprised John Oxford, whose back was to us. When he turned around, with hands clenched, and arms shaking, he stammered, 'You can't be here. You didn't register.'

'That's right,' I said calmly. I reminded him, 'I had said that I was coming, though.'

To regain his composure, he turned away from us and pointed at a large white dome, built to celebrate the millennium, in Canary Wharf. 'Have you seen the dome? Perhaps you should go downstairs and have breakfast, I'll join you in a minute.' It was obvious that he needed some time to deal with my arrival.

Robert and I went downstairs. About ten minutes later, John joined us. This time, his opening words were, 'You've created a real glitch by not registering. If you are here to talk about Spitsbergen, you are not welcome.'

'I, like everyone else, will be paying for the conference.'

'Good, good. Do you want dinner tickets for the Imperial War Museum? That costs extra.'

'Yes, that'll be fine.' John's words didn't sink in – dinner at a war museum. It was four days past Remembrance Day and a day past the Sunday commemoration in Britain of the war's ending, and John had arranged for a dinner among the paraphernalia and equipment of war.

Still waiting for the conference to begin, I told John that I was very angry and for the next 15 minutes explained why. I had my husband sit beside me as a witness. I explained that I was there to gain recognition for Norway, the team, and my project.

'I had a fax from you that said the conference was not about Spitsbergen.'

He repeated, 'If you are here to talk about Spitsbergen, you are not welcome.'

'Alan received a fax from Rod in the past few days, and Rod is going to talk about our results at this conference.'

'Oh?' he said.

I explained that it was outrageous that the team had not been kept informed of the results. Presenting the results before telling Norway and before returning the country's samples was stealing from Norway and constituted academic piracy. John shouted, 'The team won't get results because Mill Hill is paying and therefore the team is not entitled to the results.' He was saying that the results belonged to Mill Hill – NIMR – not to the team. Therefore our contribution counted for nothing. Mill Hill had the samples, Mill Hill had what it wanted. He added that Rob Webster had been pushing for the conference – the same Rob Webster, whom I had faxed repeatedly so that he and USAMRIID would not be cut out of the project, now felt free, with his colleagues, to cut out Norway and me. I added that we had verbally agreed that any laboratory that wanted to examine the samples would do so at its own cost, and that the results were the team's, not the labs'. I said that that had been decided at the team's very first meeting in Windsor (23–24 August 1996), long before he and Sir John were even involved in the project. Moreover, we all agreed in Mill Hill (3 February 1998), Toronto, and Longyearbyen to have the lab undertaking the work pay for the analyses, but that the team as a whole would own the results.

I then asked, 'What are the bone and tooth samples yielding?

'I don't know.'

'I don't believe you.' I had been tipped off that John would work with Necropolis to exhume a 1918 victim from Labrador whose body had been shipped back to England and buried there following the pandemic. There was likely to be little soft tissue – certainly less than in our supposedly poor samples – if the body had been buried in warm English soil. But there would probably be bone and tooth. I suspected that NIMR had analysed our samples of bone and tooth. I suspected that there were indeed results from these hard tissues. I asked, 'Why are you going to exhume in England?' There was no response.

'John, I know that there is going to be a press conference tomorrow.' Again, no response. 'I want to be present at it to get credit for Norway and my team. You are not to be trusted with giving credit where credit is due.'

I asked John about the media alert. He told me that he knew nothing about it. I told him what the PR company's release said. 'I have it with me. I can show it to you.'

'I'm not into that. I'm not interested.'

I accused John of deriding the samples, deriding the project, and deriding me to authors – Pete Davies and Gina Kolata – and to any member of the press who would listen. I then said, 'Despite your complaining [about the 'poor quality of the samples'], you tried to steal the results the first opportunity that you had.' He said that he felt bad for his comments to Davies and Kolata.

I replied, 'Then you should make it right. You should take back your comments in public. You've attempted character assassination.'

At this point, we were interrupted. John stopped to hug and kiss a woman who, he later explained to us, was Dr Johan Hultin's wife. John was trying to work with Johan in exhuming victims of the 1889 flu in Russia. 'It's a bit tricky getting records, though. We had wanted 1918 but were reminded a revolution was on in Russia.'

'I know, John. Perhaps you remember that I tried searching in Russia too.'

John said that we must stop arguing. I pointed out that he had said outrageous and slanderous things about me. He told me that he was embarrassed by what he had said. He apologized. I said that he had called me a 'megalomaniac and control freak' to author Pete Davies and that he 'should set the record straight in print.'

He vehemently denied calling me either. However, Pete Davies, who was invited at no cost to Oxford's conference, confirmed (verbally) that Oxford had indeed called me both.

'John, I have never said disparaging things against you. I have never spoken out against any of you. I, unlike you, have my dignity.'

'I know.'

'John, I think you blame me for your being barred from the tent. I wasn't part of it.'

'I know. I'm sorry. I'm not proud of what I have said.'

I told John that I was glad that everything was out in the open and that he understood why I was upset. He said, 'You should not be angry. I am not angry.'

'I am! I am afraid that you have no right to be. Norway was left out, and the team was left out.'

He said, 'The team could have come.'

'Some team members were not invited. Also, the team was not alerted that "Professor Oxford and his team" would be releasing the results of their hard work. John, I'm here to set the record straight. If Norway and the team are not thanked and given their proper recognition, I will stand up and give credit where credit is due at your scientific conference. Do I make myself clear?'

He nodded.

The conversation was over. John had to prepare for his opening remarks of his First International Scientific Conference. We went upstairs to seat ourselves for the day.

Rob Webster approached me. 'You've won me some money.' He

knew that I would not go down without a fight – that is, I would indeed show up to obtain proper recognition for Norway and my team.

My husband, Robert, asked him with whom he had wagered. Rob laughed, and I answered, 'Professor Oxford.' Rob just laughed, and Robert said, 'I hope that you have more success getting your money than we do.'

Noel Roberts, Roche's representative on the team, then came by. 'Very exciting, very exciting.'

I asked, 'Is it? I wouldn't know. I have yet to be informed what the results are.' Noel stared blankly at me. There was no point in telling him anything; he was after all a personal friend of Oxford's, and had clearly sided with him when Tom threatened to pull out of the project a few weeks before to the expedition.

We excused ourselves; the conference was starting. Four members of my team would speak at the conference: Rob Webster, Sir John Skehel, Rod Daniels, and John Oxford. John Oxford had organized the conference and had the backing of Sir John and Rob Webster. The three had been alerted that I was upset regarding the conference, as my faxes to John Oxford had been sent to the other two as well. They wanted to announce the results – regardless of our team's publishing agreement.

First, Ann Reid, work partner of Dr Jeffrey Taubenberger's, spoke on the Spanish influenza pandemic of 1918. She discussed the Armed Forces Institute of Pathology's characterization of the virus based on lung-tissue samples, which were fixed in formalin and embedded in paraffin, and on samples from a victim buried in the permafrost in Alaska.[1]

Next Rob Webster spoke of the transmission of avian influenza viruses to humans in Hong Kong. In the influenza outbreak of 1997, 6 of 18 infected humans died of H5N1 influenza virus, which originated from poultry markets and was transmitted directly to humans. It was eradicated by killing all the poultry in Hong Kong.[1]

At the mid-morning break, Robert and I quickly found Rod. I asked him what he was going to say. He asked whether I had received his fax regarding his planned presentation of results. I had not, but everyone else had, the working day before the conference. He said, 'Kirsty, don't blame me. I'm only doing what I'm told.'

Rod explained, 'In my defence, I am not a member of the SAG. I am not privy to what goes on, John Skehel is a member.' He was hiding behind Sir John. Not good enough. 'I was not comfortable with John Oxford's original title for the conference: "Reconstructing the 1918 Virus," so I had it changed.'

I asked what his talk was now called. He said, 'A Genetic Perspective of the 1889 and 1918 Pandemics.'

I asked, 'Are you still presenting our team's results?' He said, 'Yes. But I wrote to everyone on the team and told them what I was presenting.' Telling us the last business day before the conference did not make his actions right and gave us no time to stop him. I assumed that Rod was no longer concerned about information being 'leaked to the media,' and his not being able to publish in prestigious journals. But what about the rest of the team's publishing?

Rod knew the rules of academic publishing – namely, no previous media exposure. Perhaps Rod would have argued that presenting preliminary results at an academic conference is usually acceptable. Doing so, however, at a press conference the following day would not be.

I asked what else he knew of our results. Rod said that there was much more information that he was not presenting and that he should have the whole virus sequenced within the year. I told him of John's press release. For the first time, Rod showed some regret. He was clearly shocked. His friend John Oxford was taking credit for Rod's analyses of our samples. He said, 'You're kidding.' We offered to show the media alert to him, but the conference resumed.

I quickly instructed, 'Rod, you must give credit where credit is due. You must thank Norway, and you must thank each member of the research team and recognize what each person accomplished.' He agreed.

'Rod, if you don't, I will stand up and set the record straight.' These words were becoming my mantra. 'Rod, I told John Oxford the same thing.'

At lunch, Ann Reid asked if she could sit with me. I nodded, even though I knew the disparaging remarks that she and Jeffrey Taubenberger had made – how they wanted to be seen as separate from the 'showy Spitsbergen expedition.' Ann told me that John wanted to work with Taubenberger and her. Was she asking me my opinion? John wanted to work not only with Johan Hultin, but also with Taubenberger and Ann. He was clearly cultivating their friendship. It is not likely that they were aware of his previous outbursts against Taubenberger at our Mill Hill and Toronto meetings.

Johan Hultin then asked if he could join us. He was very gracious to me, congratulating me on my work. I could not say that I admired his work. I thought his not asking the state authorities permission to undertake the work and his not taking any safety precautions irresponsible. I spoke to him about what I did admire – the fact that he had climbed Mt Everest. Ann jumped in, 'Yes, the more you know of Johan, the more remarkable he is.' I excused myself. I found it difficult to make small talk. I left – only to bump into one of the co-producers of Elliot Halpern's documentary, and author Pete Davies. Pete asked if I had read his book.[2] I had not. He asked what I was doing in London. The results of the team's work and seven years of my work were to be announced by 'John Oxford and his team,' and they wondered what I was 'doing in London.' I explained that John was releasing the results of my team's project and that I was there to ensure credit for all involved. Both men stood still. I said, 'John is attempting academic piracy.'

Pete said, 'Oh, Kirsty, we know. We all know what you've been up against.' What did he mean? Was he siding with me, despite disparaging remarks (according to Tom Bergan) in his book? Tom, who had read the piece, said Pete had libelled me and that I should sue him.

Pete said, 'I am on your side; you should read my book. I am clearly on your side.'

At this point Sir John interrupted the conversation. He casually asked, 'Are you here on vacation?' Seven years of my work being exposed to all and sundry, and Sir John asked if I were 'here on vacation'! I did not answer, and he walked away. These were the only words that he spoke to me throughout the conference.

In the afternoon, Rod spoke on the 'Genetic Perspective of the 1889 and 1918 Pandemics.' I learned more about my team's results. There was a real buzz in the room; Ann Reid could be seen writing down all the details. Rod presented brand new information, never before known, about the deadliest outbreak of disease in recorded history. Short fragments of the 1918 Spanish flu virus were recovered from the lung, liver, kidney, and brain. This suggested that in some victims, the virus had spread from the lungs, via the bloodstream, to other organs. It did not attack just the lungs, as had been thought. Virus fragments found in the brain perhaps lent support to the theory that the Spanish flu of 1918 and the killer of the 1920s, encephalitis lethargica, truly were related.

The fragment sequences differed from those in the cases reported by

Dr Taubenberger and Ann Reid in the United States. The differences suggested that perhaps the 1918 pandemic may have involved more than one virus. Rod explained that more results were expected.

Rod noted, 'There is a young lady in the audience who kinda got the ball rolling in Longyearbyen.' He then showed a slide with all my team members' names and briefly described each person's contribution. And there was a final note at the bottom of the slide thanking Norway. Excellent!

I should have been happy. After all, the project that I initiated was providing answers to one of the past century's greatest medical mysteries, and Norway and my team had been acknowledged. But I felt sadness, anger, and bitterness, as my Norwegian and Canadian team members were not present to hear the news for themselves. I planned to answer for Norway and my missing team members at the press conference – John's gala event following the scientific conference on Tuesday afternoon.

At the end of the first day's proceedings, I noticed Rob Webster and a woman arguing over a sheet of paper. I guessed that it was something for the media. The media always seemed to bring out the passion in some of my team.

After Rob left, I asked if the paper was the press release. The woman snatched it from the table and shoved it behind her back. She said, 'You can't see it.'

I said, 'I don't think you know who I am. My name is Dr Duncan. I am the project leader of the Spitsbergen expedition.'

'I know.'

'I would like to see the press release, particularly if the information pertains to my team.'

'I'll have to ask Professor Oxford.'

Many minutes passed. Eventually, the woman escorted John from the conference. John said, 'Of course, Kirsty can see the release, but it is not ready.' It was ready. The woman was holding it in her hand. 'If you and your husband go for a twenty-minute walk, it will be ready when you get back.' Had John forgotten the morning's conversation? Had he forgotten that I already had a copy of the press release issued by the PR company the previous Friday (Figure 17)?

Robert and I disappeared down the steps and out the door of the hotel. We phoned home to update everyone. I said to my father, 'They wouldn't dare write a new release when I have the old one, would

---

Influenza: Past, Present and Future
Press briefing
Tuesday, 15 November 1999

Who:

- Chairman Professor John Oxford, virologist and influenza pathogenicity expert (Royal London Hospital, UK) will provide the first media update on the results of the Spitzbergen expedition together with an historical perspective on influenza and the key lessons learnt since the Pandemic of 1918. – *A retrospective look at influenza – what have we learnt?*

- Professor Rob Webster, (St Judes Children's Research Hospital, USA), leading virology and molecular biology expert will provide an overview on the composition of the virus and how changes in the composition have, in the past, hampered the development of an effective flu treatment which targets viral replication – *Understanding the ever changing influenza virus*

- Professor Claude Hannoun (of the Institut Pasteur) expert in influenza and respiratory viruses, presents on the annual implications, direct and indirect, of influenza on society, business, commerce and primary care. – *The burden of influenza in today's world*

 ➢ (GP from Switzerland) will give a practical insight into the burden of influenza and provide an update on the Swiss experience of Tamiflu in this flu season

- Professor Frederick Hayden, leading virologist, (University of Virginia School of Medicine, USA) will present on the development of neuraminidase inhibitors in influenza management, focussing on oseltamivir (Tamiflu™) and discussing its role in influenza treatment for the new millennium - *Consolidating lessons learnt: what the future holds for sufferers of influenza*

Why:

- The symposium will provide the first opportunity to hear the data from the Spitzbergen expedition undertaken by Professor Oxford and his team.

- The new oral neuraminidase inhibitor, oseltamivir phosphate (Tamiflu). Tamiflu was approved in Switzerland on 20 September 1999 and other approvals are expected imminently.

- World leading virologists and influenza experts will put recent developments in influenza treatment in to context, focussing on the following:
  - Influenza through the ages
  - Challenge of dealing with the ever-changing influenza virus
  - Influenza management in primary care setting

- Lunch will be provided for journalists prior to the press briefing

Where: "The Classroom" at the London Aquarium, County Hall, Riverside Building, Westminster Bridge Road, London, SE1 7PB

When: Tuesday, 15 November 1999

they?' He gave his stock answer, 'Kirsty, they all have their own agendas. You'd better get back.'

When we returned, I was indeed presented with a brand new press release (Figure 18). It now read, 'the symposium will provide the first opportunity to hear the data from 1918 expeditions ... Details will be presented of a new international expedition which is planning to probe back even further to the 1889 influenza pandemic.'

There was no longer any mention of 'Professor Oxford and his team.' I told the woman that that was not the original press release. I told her that she was lying, and I took out Friday's alert. She said that Friday's release was an old media alert. I said that we obtained the release from the PR company for the conference the previous working day. The BBC later confirmed that the Friday release was the press release that it had received.

Torsten Hoof, the funder from Roche, hearing the disturbance, kindly came over and introduced himself to me. I could not contain my anger any longer. I told him that Oxford was committing academic piracy and that I was present to set the record straight on behalf of Norway and my team. Torsten asked what I wanted. I said that I needed to speak at the press conference the next day. He said that he would discuss the next day's business with me the next morning.

At 6:30 p.m., two coaches arrived to transport delegates from the hotel to the Imperial War Museum for the evening function. Walking through the museum's door, Robert and I were appalled to see dinner tables set out amid tanks, submarines, and warheads; planes hung from the ceiling above the tables. John and his wife, Gillian, greeted their arriving guests and explained the significance of the venue – 1918, the year of Spanish flu and the last year of war.

We should have left right then. Remembrance Day had just passed. Dr Howard Phillips, a South African historian who had hosted a meeting on Spanish flu the previous year, was equally distressed. He said, 'I am surprised that John would host a dinner here. It is in poor taste.' Robert and I stopped to phone Tanya Talaga from the *Toronto Star*, and then we were ushered to our tables.

We were placed behind a bus, at the last table, in the back of the great hall. John's very close friends were sitting on either side of Robert and me, and Esther Oxford, her back to a missile, was sitting two seats from Robert. John later explained to Robert that he 'seated members of

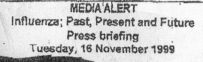

MEDIA ALERT
Influenza: Past, Present and Future
Press briefing
Tuesday, 16 November 1999

- **Chairman Professor John Oxford** (Royal London Hospital, UK) virologist and influenza pathogenicity expert will provide an update of the 1918 pandemic, information on an outbreak in France and the UK in 1916, together with an historical perspective on influenza and the key lessons learnt.
  – A retrospective look at influenza – what have we learnt?

- **Professor Robert Webster**, (St Judes Children's Research Hospital, USA) leading virology and molecular biology expert will give an overview on the composition of the virus and how changes in the composition have, in the past, hampered the development of an effective flu treatment which targets viral replication
  – Understanding the ever changing influenza virus

- **Professor Claude Hannoun** (Institute Pasteur, France) expert in influenza and respiratory viruses, presents on the annual implications, direct and indirect, of influenza on society, business and commerce as well as complications that can result from influenza.
  – The burden of influenza in today's world
- **Dr Thomas Aeschbach** (Lausanne, Switzerland) will give a practical insight into the burden of influenza and provide an update on how the new treatments will impact on influenza in Switzerland this year.

- **Professor Frederick Hayden** (University of Virginia School of Medicine, USA) leading virologist, will present on the development of neuraminidase inhibitors in influenza management, and discuss their role in influenza treatment for the new millennium – *Consolidating lessons learnt: what the future holds for sufferers of influenza*

- The symposium will provide the first opportunity to hear the data from 1918 expeditions. Did this massive outbreak start earlier in 1916 in France?
- Details will be presented of a new international expedition which is planning to probe back even further to the 1889 influenza pandemic.
- Data will be presented on the new oral neuraminidase inhibitor, oseltamivir (Tamiflu) which was approved in Switzerland on 20 September 1999. Other approvals are expected imminently.
- World leading virologists and influenza experts will put recent developments in influenza treatment in to context, focussing on the following:
  - Influenza through the ages
  - Challenge of dealing with the ever-changing influenza virus
  - Influenza management in primary care setting

- Lunch will be provided for journalists prior to the press briefing

"The Classroom" at the London Aquarium, County Hall, Riverside Building, Westminster Bridge Road, London. SE1 7PB

Tuesday, 16 November 1999 at 13.30 – 16.00

Figure 18 John Oxford's modified release, 15 November 1999.

my family or staff at each of the tables for hospitality.' Or for damage control, perhaps?

I ignored Esther. I talked with the man next to me – a runner and a pilot. We talked about racing, and we talked about flying. Then, out of the blue, Esther asked what everyone thought of her article.

Robert responded. 'Esther, your article couldn't help but remind me of the task we were assigned in grade school at the start of each new year, to write, 'What I did on my Summer Vacation with Mommy and Daddy.'

Esther looked away. Robert continued, 'You knew the project was Kirsty's.'

'I was biased from the beginning ... I was determined to see my father succeed.' Esther looked off into the distance with tears in her eyes.

The speeches were starting. The talks were followed by one of John's crew singing the 'Influenza Blues,' the only song written at the time, John believed, about the 1918 flu. The woman's voice resonated through the great halls and echoed through the artillery.

The singing was to be followed by a live band and dance. 'Robert,' I whispered, 'I'm not going to be part of a dance in a mausoleum. Let's go.' We made our excuses and left the building.

We had no sleep following the dinner. I began calling Alan, Charles, and Peter to fill them in. I could not reach Tom, as he was on a business trip; I would have to wait for him to contact me.

A fax from reporter Maryn McKenna was slipped under our hotel-room door. Robert read: 'I am pleased to hear that there are viral samples and I am appalled at the behaviour of some members of the team – and I am so glad to hear that you flew over there and muscled your way into their press conference.' After Robert had read these kind words, I returned messages and prepared for the next day's battle.

Conference: Day Two

On Tuesday morning, 16 November, I watched Rod Daniels give an interview to the BBC. Afterwards, I asked the interviewer if Rod had discussed the results and what press release the reporters had been given. Rod had indeed discussed the team's results, despite his earlier fear of information being leaked to the media. The BBC had received the release about 'Professor Oxford and his team' – not the one newly prepared in the minutes in which Robert and I were told to walk. The

BBC reporter asked why I wanted to know. I briefly explained the seven-year project and what had transpired since Thursday. Wednesday seemed a lifetime ago.

He said, 'That's incredible. Would you be willing to do an interview with us?'

'I can't. I promised to give the funder of the conference the opportunity to make it right for Norway and the team. I have to wait to see what he says.'

When the funding agent – Torsten – and I met, he again asked me what I wanted. Robert waited by my side as a witness.

'I want to speak at the press conference to set the record straight.'

'It is not possible. Your speaking has not been arranged.'

'Then arrange it.'

'May I suggest that you write a number of points and Professor Oxford could present them at the conference.'

'I do not want Professor Oxford talking about my team's project. He attempted academic piracy. He won't credit the team.'

'Kirsty, I give you my word that John will give credit where credit is due.'

'No one can make John do anything. He does what he likes; he is not easily handled. He makes promises and he breaks them.'

'Kirsty, I give you my word.'

At this point Robert jumped in. He said, 'I guess that you as the funder would have some control over John, especially if John wants funding on future projects.'

Torsten laughed and repeated, 'I give you my word.'

'Torsten, if John does not do the right thing, I will stand up and set the record straight.'

'Kirsty, you must not make a scene. It is our first conference. We want it to continue.'

'Torsten, I have never made a scene. I have been a lady throughout this whole ugly mess. I suggest, however, that you see to it that John does the right thing today.'

'I will, I will.'

'Thank you.' I then wrote out six points for John to read: 'Dr. Kirsty Duncan is the project leader, who began the project seven years ago. Professor Tom Bergan is the Norwegian co-ordinator for the project. The tissue samples, collected safely and ethically, are yielding good results. Dr. Rod Daniels, National Institute for Medical Research, has been performing the analyses. The project was a team effort and the results are a team success. [John had to recognize each member of the team.] Finally, the team is very grateful to the community of Longyearbyen and the people of Svalbard and Norway.'

Robert and I then left the conference. I declined the BBC interview, as Torsten had given me his word. The BBC said, 'If they don't make good on their word, please do the interview.'

Following the agreement, we were picked up by a Canadian television station with an office in London for which I had agreed to do an interview. Little did I know that Tanya's stories[3-5] had given me the backing of the Canadian media and Canadians from whom I received numerous wonderful, encouraging letters.

The Canadian reporters drove me to the conference. 'We are here to follow you around. You do what you have to.' I explained Torsten's promises and hoped that there would not be a scene.

Prior to John's press conference, I again spoke with him. This time I had no witness. I once again explained how angry I was. I said that he had to credit Norway and the team.

John was trapped. The funding agent had ordered that he do the right thing – that is, acknowledge that the project was a seven-year undertaking, a team effort, that every member's contribution was necessary and important, and that Norway was central to the project. And I sat, glaring, mouth pursed, and arms crossed, in the front row of the press conference. He had no way out.

John bent over backwards to credit Norway, the team, and me with the excellent findings. He spoke graciously about the project and the team and elaborated on my six points, which had been made into a slide and were presented on the screen. All team members (a slide showed their names and affiliations) and their roles were also recognized.

He had recognized Norway, he had recognized my team! I had come to London for these two things, and they had actually happened! After he spoke, I walked over and thanked him.

But I could not forget that:

- He had not invited me to a conference releasing the results of my expedition.
- He had excluded the members of the team of the host country – Norway.
- He had not allowed me to speak of the expedition.

- He had chosen to release the team's results without permission from the team.
- By informing the media, he had threatened the team's opportunity to publish in refereed scientific journals.
- He did not correct the original media alert of 'Professor Oxford and his team,' which was distributed throughout Europe.

Rod Daniels, Rob Webster, and I then proceeded to the stage to entertain questions from among the one hundred gathered journalists. There was a question on flu followed by a Canadian reporter asking John why the Canadian scientists had been left out of the conference.

I was surprised that several Canadian journalists were present. All the press tags were European; there were, however, no Norwegian tags. John briefly answered, 'This is a virology conference.'

The Canadians were not about to let matters drop. Another reporter said that John's answer was not good enough and asked again why the Canadians were left out. John panicked and said, 'Perhaps Dr Duncan can answer that.' I made it very clear that I was pleased that 'Things had been righted – today.' They questioned me further, and I explained the history of the past week.

I heard Rob Webster mutter, 'Oh, shit.' It was unfortunate that politics and jealousies overshadowed the release of the excellent results. However, the press asked me, and I gave the truth.

Following the questioning, the journalists swarmed me. Apparently, the swarming is called a 'scrum.' I had never experienced anything like it in my life – microphones shoved in my face; bright lights, I couldn't see anything. And then Robert, beaming, winking, and mouthing that I had done it. I had got credit for everyone.

While I was swarmed, apparently so too was John Oxford, who kept repeating, in response to all the questions about the absence of Norway, the absence of the project leader, and academic piracy, 'It was a virology conference,' and 'I'm not into that.'

I was exhausted. I wanted to go home – not back to the hotel, but home – to Toronto. Dr Johan Hultin came up to me. He wanted to share a glass of wine with me to say congratulations. I explained that I do not drink, and so Robert rushed off to get me a glass of my substitute orange juice. Johan was acting like a gentleman.

As I was leaving, I saw Rob Webster. I said that I was sorry that the story had come out in such a fashion. Unbelievably, he said, 'You've got to step out of the limelight. It is Rod's turn.'

I said, 'Rob, I didn't do this for the media. This was a very expensive undertaking. I did it for Norway and the team. You tried to cut Norway and the team out.'

He said, 'Oh, come on, you love it. We all love it. This is why we do it.'

'Rob, we have the MOU. You folks couldn't release the results without the whole team agreeing.'

'The MOU is dead. You didn't sign the extension.'

(The project was to 'terminate on the earlier of October, 1999, or one calendar year following commencement of Phase II.' As the termination date approached, St Jude Children's Research Hospital produced an extension to the original MOU. Prior to signing, I spoke with my lawyer, who warned me not to sign until all other SAG members did so. Thus I would assure that everyone was bound to the agreement; therefore no one could publish the team's results without prior agreement by the SAG. If someone refused to sign, I too would not sign. I would then be free to 'set the record straight' should anyone try to release the results.)

'My lawyer was looking into my signing, but a number of promises had to be met first. For example, John Oxford had to sign. I was afraid that if he didn't sign, he would try to do just what he has done – steal the results. Besides, Tom, Alan, John Skehel and you had signed.'

'John Skehel never signed.'

'That's not what your institution told me. Your institution put me on hold during my phone call, looked up the agreement, and told me that only John Oxford and I hadn't signed.'

Rob repeated, 'John Skehel didn't sign.' Now things made sense. Earlier, I didn't believe that Sir John, as director of NIMR, would dare to break the team's MOU by releasing results.

Then I asked, 'Are you happy with the results?'

He said that he was thrilled. He said, 'You wonderful, wonderful girl.' He stated to my husband that he had respect for me.

I asked him about whether he was going to do any of the PCR work. He said 'no.' I asked about USAMRIID. Apparently, that was not going to happen either. He did not elaborate.

'Rob, why didn't you respond to my three faxes about PCR then?'

'I never got them.'

'I faxed them to your assistant. She was going to get them to you in Hong Kong. They were marked "urgent."'

Despite his praise of me to my husband, two minutes later he spoke with the press. 'The problem is that some people don't want to give up their place at the centre of the stage. It's time to let the scientists take over.'

Tom, Bjorn, and I had not been invited to the 'release of the results.' And if the British media had not tipped me off, Norway and many team members would not have been recognized.

But I had managed to get credit for everyone involved. But would I be able to get credit for the team in the future? Would I receive updates of results? Would Norway receive its promised samples for bacteriology? Would Canada's BSL 4 laboratory be ready, and would Canada receive its samples for PCR? Would another laboratory replicate Rod Daniel's findings? And when would the team publish the results in academic journals?

It was impossible to answer any of these questions. My hunch, however, was that getting information out of Britain, and returning the samples to Norway, would continue to be difficult, if not impossible.

18 Sharing Samples?

November 1999–November 2000

Following the London conference of 15–16 November 1999, I continued to fight for information on our developing results, and I continued to fight for Canada's samples. The samples finally arrived in 2000.

While waiting for results from Britain, I heard from a Canadian scientist (who insisted on anonymity) that the rumour from the Armed Forces Institute of Pathology (AFIP) – Dr Taubenberger's outfit – was that my team made up the results announced in England. The Canadian also reported that 'others are now examining the link between Spanish flu and encephalitis lethargica.'

More Results, March–April 2000

By late March 2000, I still had received no news from London. On the 27th, I wrote to Sir John: 'I would be most grateful for an update on the analyses of the Svalbard samples, as the team has not had any information since November (1999) when Rod provided team members with information prior to giving his talk at "Influenza – Past, Present and Future: Genetics of Virulence and Pathogenicity."'

On 29 March, Rod Daniels faxed Tom Bergan the requested information. 'I am now in a position to put a complete HA (haemagglutinin gene) together from brain 1, have all but the coding region for the C-terminal end of HA2 from another and about half from a third. Since November, I have started to look for fragments (and have a few) from four other genes (NP, NA, MA, NS) but most of these still require sequencing. ... I understand you (and others) may think things are progressing slowly but it is painstaking, soul-destroying work to be putting this thing together from such small fragments (if we had a virus it would have been done in under a month).' He had sent samples to the Winnipeg lab which had a large team of people for the work. 'We are in e-mail discussion and I have given them practical support in terms of supplying lists of the primers I have designed for the project and modifications I have made to the RT-PCR process. If they can independently provide a small amount of sequence information which matches my HA data I think we will be in a position to publish. They are also considering what to do in terms of looking for bacteria and performing histologic studies.' He had not been in touch 'with the non-English members of the team since November. I don't know if this is related to some of the "un-truths" that appeared in the Canadian press around the time of the November conference.'

I could have predicted Rod's letter. Like other letters from NIMR, the fax appeared helpful, as if Rod was sharing new information. Rod had told my husband, Robert, and me his newly faxed information in November. Nothing was new. What was nice to hear, however, was that NIMR appeared to be working with the Canadian lab. I had to laugh at Rod's mentioning 'un-truths.' Clearly, he had not read the Canadian press closely enough, or he would have read Tom's comments regarding British 'untruths' and Tom's being left out of the conference.

Rod faxed me on 6 April. 'Attached is a fairly detailed summary of what has happened since November 1999. Things have moved on considerably, not least in terms of the phylogenetic analyses performed with the HA sequences.' Rod elaborated: 'Since November 1999, PCR rescues of influenza gene fragments have been pursued from brain specimens only (as these have proven better than other organs in terms of fragment recovery). For HA, as fragments, we now have a complete sequence from brain 7, all but the C-terminal coding region for HA2 from brain 1, and a third brain (6) is yielding fragments currently. From these studies, it does appear that there are foci of infection/influenza presence in the brains as not all extracts from individual brains have yielded results. ... The sequences from brains 1 and 7 are clearly related but they differ from one another. Phylogenetic analysis shows them to map in a clade with the "early" human H1 viruses.' He and his colleagues had 'designed, and had synthesized, sets of primers to attempt generation of four other influenza genes (NP, NA, MA, NS). The success of generating fragments for the other four genes has been lower than for HA.'

The Canadians, Rod continued, wrote that they 'would start extracting RNA and use the HA gene and the British primer design to evaluate their PCR procedures. Once HA amplification works we will continue amplification of the M and eventually NA segments. All this could be done in collaboration; at least we would favour that very much. What has been done in respect to bacteria? Has someone looked into this more closely already? If not we would be interested to start something using PCR approaches.'

As for bacterial studies, the British had responded that 'nothing has been done. I have done quite a bit of background reading regarding what was isolated in 1918 but there was no "single" bacterium that stands out – lots of different things were isolated and this may reflect to some extent what particular researchers were looking for. The one interesting pointer we have come across is that Haemophilus influenzae used to exist in non-capsulated and capsulated forms but today only the capsulated form is found – how might one probe for this using PCR?'

I now had some new information: which brain material had yielded results, what these results were, and what the Canadians were willing to analyse. There was also more evidence that the British wanted to work openly with the Canadians. I was very pleased.

Returning Team Member? Norway's Samples?
April–November 2000

On 11 April, I received probably one of the most shocking faxes of the whole eight-year project. Sir John wrote: 'As some of you already know, Rod Daniels has completed the sequence of one gene for haemagglutinin from the Svalbard samples and almost completed another. They are closely related and clearly early H1 haemagglutinin. They are a little different from the sequences published by Reid, Fanning, Hultin, and Taubenberger, and as a consequence we would like to ... confirm the data. Simply, would the same sequences be obtained if parallel tissue samples were analyzed independently elsewhere?' Skehel wanted to work with Taubenberger's laboratory 'because of their expertise and commitment to the topic. As a consequence I have contacted Jeffrey Taubenberger by telephone and he would be pleased to be involved in a blind analysis of parallel samples. Obviously, in my view, this seems to be an excellent outcome. He understands that nothing will be sent to him without the agreement of the SAG and we should now discuss this matter.'

NIMR wanted to involve Dr Taubenberger, who had worked behind the team's back. Moreover, John Skehel had previously said of him, 'So let him go. We don't need him. We can certainly do the work ourselves.' Furthermore, information was still being shared with the virologists before the project leader. The fax, though addressed to me, had started, 'As some of you already know.'

I responded immediately and copied my correspondence to the entire SAG. 'I find your fax of April 11th, 2000 most distressing. You and your lab have been entrusted with Norway's and the team's samples. However, you operate as if the samples are yours alone. How could you contact Dr. Taubenberger without discussing the matter with the team first? The *team* decided at Mill Hill in February, 1998, to let Dr. Taubenberger work on his own, after he had secretly worked with Dr. Hultin – despite his being a member of the Spitsbergen expedition.' I went again through the tortuous break-up and Taubenberger's denigration of the project. 'Why would you call someone, who has, time and again, put down the team's work? On behalf of the team, I must ask you to put in writing that no samples will be sent to Dr. Taubenberger. Please respect the team's wishes.'

Moreover, I was unwilling to exploit Taubenberger for our own purposes. 'If you were prepared to ship samples to Dr. Taubenberger, perhaps testing for live virus is now complete, and you could now return Norway's samples? Or perhaps Dr. Taubenberger was going to work at USAMRIID's BSL 4 lab, as Dr. Webster was to have done. If this is the case, surely Dr. Webster should have the opportunity before Dr. Taubenberger.' 'The Canadian lab should be involved in attempting replication ... The samples are in Canada. The Canadian lab wants to work in a collegial manner with you. I am sure that you appreciate that the Canadian lab is more than capable of undertaking a "blind analysis of parallel samples."'

I continued: 'This is not the first time that you have acted in a less-than-open manner. After promising repeatedly to update both Tom and me regarding the team's results, you allowed your employee (I do not want Rod put in a compromising position!) to release the team's results at an academic conference, followed by a press conference. This was most discouraging, as (1) both Tom and I had been assured by you that "whenever there is anything" (re. the results) to tell the SAG, you "will do so with pleasure"; and (2) Rod was most concerned that "if too much is leaked to the media, from whatever source, that it could prevent us from publishing in prestigious journals." The fact that Rod

wrote to the team one business day before the conference does not justify any of your actions. Please abide by the agreements under which
we have been working.'

Needless to say, there was no response to my fax. On 19 April, I
again faxed Sir John: 'You asked for a prompt response to your April
11th, 2000 fax. I would ask that you return the favour and promptly
put in writing that no samples will be sent to Dr. Taubenberger, as he
has acted dishonourably towards the team.'

Tom faxed Sir John on the 28th: 'I will not repeat the reasons and reasoning, but it was clearly a consensus when we met at Mill Hill in 1998
that he (Dr. Taubenberger) should not be included.' And the Canadian
and Norwegian facilities were waiting for samples.

> Consequently, it would seem that asking Taubenberger now is not to be
> recommended. If he were asked to process our samples, clearly, a new
> consensus would have to be sought. Kirsty is not in favour. I have not
> been convinced that it is a good idea to change our policy.
>
> Comments made in two recently published books and ascribed to Dr.
> Taubenberger is also consistent with the above.
>
> Conceivably, recent developments indicate that Mill Hill would like to
> call for Dr. Taubenberger's assistance.
>
> However, we have other laboratories close to our group, e.g. the Cana-
> dian laboratory which has received specimens. They should be both will-
> ing and qualified to help out?
>
> Another question that we would like is that specimens for processing of
> bacterial queries should be returned to Norway. We have a BSL 3 unit at
> Professor Berdal's department in Oslo. Since no viable virus has been
> found in the specimens at Mill Hill, there should be no security reason for
> not distributing the specimens to us. Of course, one might run out of
> material to decipher the viral genome. If that is so, it should be stated so
> that all involved may help to solve the problem. We would particularly
> like one of the teeth and lung and intestinal samples.

On 2 May, Alan Heginbottom wrote to John Skehel. In bold letters, he
stated: '**At this time I am not persuaded that it is appropriate to share
samples with Taubenberger.**'

> Before contemplating the sharing of samples with Taubenberger, I think a
> better effort should be made to work through the analysis plans to which
> we had all agreed prior to the actual exhumations taking place.

Furthermore, I am concerned over what biological safety levels will be applied. My understanding is that Taubenberger does not have access to a BSL 4 lab. Thus, any samples sent to him would, I presume, be handled under BSL 3 or lower conditions. If the samples can indeed be handled under these lower levels of safety, then surely there are other labs and other workers who could undertake replicate analyses, rather than involve Taubenberger.

Finally, as soon as the samples can be handled at a BSL 3 or lower level of safety, you must provide our Norwegian colleagues with a suite of tissue samples and with all the newspaper and other artifacts which were retained during the autopsies. This is, to me, both important and urgent.

I faxed Sir John again on the 11th, attaching copies of Alan and Tom's responses. 'Further to my communication to you of April 12th and April 19th, 2000, I must again ask you to put in writing that no samples will be sent to Dr. Taubenberger, as he has acted dishonourably towards the team ... The three of us do not favour sending Dr. Taubenberger the team's samples ... A clear majority has been needed to push new ideas through. At least three of the six members of the SAG are against sending the samples. There is no majority to push forward the new idea.'

There was no response to any of my requests. On 14 August, I decided to fax Sir John again. 'I am writing to you for some information, please. First, when will samples be returned to Norway? I have just learned (August 10th, 2000) from Tom that no samples have yet been returned to Norway. This is extremely embarrassing, as: (1) it is now two years since our 1998 expedition when samples were retrieved; (2) my permission required that samples be given to Norway; and (3) our team promised to work under the rules and regulations of the permission.' I added: 'Since the exhumations, you suggested that Dr. Taubenberger be allowed access to the samples. (Incidentally, I am still waiting for confirmation that no samples were sent to Dr. Taubenberger ...) Dr. Taubenberger does not have a BSL 4 lab, and we agreed that the samples could not be shipped to anything less than BSL 4 containment. If you were prepared to ship samples to Dr. Taubenberger, perhaps testing for live virus is now complete, and you could now return Norway's samples?'

Sir John responded on the 22nd: 'As you know, small pieces of all soft tissue specimens, one bone marrow and one tooth, have been screened for infectious influenza virus and found to be negative. However, as the RT-PCR detection of influenza nucleic acid has been sporadic (not all specimens from the same product yield products), we cannot categorically state that "infectious influenza virus is not present." We therefore continue to treat samples as if they might contain virus, in spite of consensus opinion that the chances of infectious virus remaining are remote. Consequently, as Tom already knows, samples can be sent to Norway at any time to a containment 4 lab (we are governed by the British HSE regulations), just as they were sent to the Canadian lab.' In response to me: 'The answer to your question regarding Dr. Taubenberger is that no samples were sent. Those discussed would have been inactivated by us, prior to release, following procedures he has described in relation to the Alaskan samples. Such inactivated samples could also be sent to Tom.' At this point, NIMR would not return the samples to Norway, as Tom did not want deactivated material for his country. And Dr Taubenberger would not have access to the team's samples.

On 4 September I thanked Sir John for his correspondence and asked four lingering questions: '(1) Who exactly is performing the analyses on the samples? ... It was my understanding that just Rod and his assistant have access to our samples. Despite this, a number of us (in Canada and Norway) continue to see that John Oxford is undertaking PCR on the Spitsbergen samples for your Institute, NIMR. (2) Is John Oxford undertaking any analyses? If so, which ones, and for which Institute? (3) Is your Institute performing only PCR and screening for live virus or are bacteriological, histological, or other tests being performed concurrently? (4) You mentioned that bone marrow and one tooth have been screened for infectious influenza virus. Has PCR been performed on bone marrow and tooth as well? If so, what are the results?'

I would fax Tom a copy and add: 'Tom, I'm asking this for your benefit. I would like J.S. to put in writing that they are not performing bacteriological studies, as Norway wanted to do this. Have you thought about what you want done about the samples? i.e. Do you want J.S. to deactivate the samples and send them to Norway, or do you want to wait for testing of live virus to be completed?'

Sir John responded on the 8th: 'Analyses are being performed by Rod Daniels (Influenza RT-PCR and attempts to isolate) and Alan Douglas (attempts to isolate), both of whom are "affiliated" with NIMR. John Oxford has not/does not have access to the samples. Samples have been sent to the containment 4 lab in Canada only, where analyses are being carried out under the auspices of Harvey Artsob (to our knowledge these are RT-PCR studies only so far). We have and continue to perform screening for live virus and influenza RT-PCR only at this time, which remains the primary objective of the project. Bacteriological, histological and "other" tests will require additional experts/ expertise. The PCR results on the bone marrow and tooth extracts were negative, but only 1 specimen of each has been looked at.'

Sir John's correspondence told me three important facts. First, despite John Oxford's claims (in the Canadian and Norwegian media) to be performing PCR, he had no access to the team's samples. Second, NIMR was not performing bacteriological and histological tests. This was good news, as Norwegian scientists and Charles Smith, respectively, wanted to do these studies. Third, one sample of bone marrow and one tooth extract were negative for virus fragments. Had other samples been tested? Was John Oxford looking for skeletal material from a Spanish flu victim buried in warm English soil? Charles and I wondered.

I had also re-established communication with the governor of Svalbard. On 14 August 2000, I wrote: 'It is two years since I have been in your beautiful and enchanting Svalbard, and two years since I have had the pleasure of talking with my friends in Longyearbyen ... Once again, I am very pleased to tell you that analyses continued to be performed on the samples.' I briefly reviewed the results released at the November 1999 conference in London and asked about the cemetery's recovery. 'I would very much like to know how the cemetery looks today. Is the ground healing? Is there a need for further clean-up? If so, we will be pleased to undertake any required work. As you know, we set aside funds should further restoration be required. I would be most grateful for a report from you.'

I did not mention Norway's samples as I did not want to embarrass my British colleagues and Tom had agreed in April 1998 at the team's Toronto meeting to return his country's samples. On 31 August 2000, I wrote privately to Tom: 'You will notice that I did not address the whereabouts of Norway's samples in my letter. Tom, please know that I have asked repeatedly for Norway's samples. I copied you my latest request on August 14th, 2000. I also copied you John Skehel's response on August 22nd. What do you want to do about the samples?' I added that a letter to the Norwegian Ministry of Health might force Sir John's hand.

Tom and I soon spoke. He did not want a letter sent, as it might initiate an international incident, and he did not want his good name besmirched.

'Tom, what do you want me to do?'

'Nothing. Nothing can be done. They'll never return the samples. It's time to stop asking. They are rogues, rogues in scientists' clothing.'

'But Tom, what about my promises?'

'You've done everything that you can. I've done everything that I can. There is no more to be done. You can't make others do anything.'

'Well Tom, do you at least want the deactivated samples?'

'No, they're no good. We wanted the same samples London got. And if we can't have them, we don't want any. ... Maybe, you could talk to Rob Webster on our behalf. Perhaps, he could talk to his good friend Sir John.'

But Tom rallied – and asked John Skehel for Norway's samples – on 30 October: 'Professor Hans Preus would like to visit you to procure the specimens we need: tooth, intestines and respiratory tract to recover bacterial traces. When would it be suitable for you to meet him?'

Rod Daniels responded on 1 November: 'As we have made clear on a number of occasions, we can send only fixed materials to Norway as the samples collected in Svalbard still have containment 4 classification. Since we have screened only small pieces of soft tissues and one tooth for presence of influenza infectious virus (all were negative) we cannot say categorically that infectious virus is not present, not to mention other agents. This is backed up by not all extracts of the same tissue being PCR positive, potentially indicating "foci of infection." In terms of sample fixation, formaldehyde is the most commonly used reagent and would be that of choice from our HSE's perspective. Let me know if Professor Hans Preus is happy to work with such fixed material or has a preferred fixation procedure. I will then arrange the fixation and transport to the required lab in Norway.' The fax was signed, 'Rod Overwhelmed and underpaid!'

Recovering Cemetery, August–November 2000

I heard from the governor of Svalbard's office on 22 August: 'We are pleased to hear from you and thankful for the information given about your project. The cemetery is recovering. Last year the grass was greener than before, but this year it is back to normal. We can still see the marks of the cutting of the turf – and it will be visible for a few years. The cemetery might, however, suffer more from increased traffic, but we hope it is not because of your project, but the increasing stream of tourists. We add a few photos to show the status just now' (Figures 19 and 20). 'With the scientific results you predict, we feel that the temporary wounds on the cemetery are small, and so far we see no need for further restoration.'

I suggested to Tom that we give the remaining money from the project to the governor's office (or another appropriate authority) in turn for its 'signing off' on clean-up of the cemetery. Should there be a problem, the authorities could respond immediately and as they saw fit.

Tom agreed, and so on 15 September I faxed John Oxford, as his budget included the contingency funds for restoration. 'I am writing to you in order to ask for your assistance. First, I need to know how much money is left from the Spitsbergen account. In fact, a complete accounting of the monies spent would very much be appreciated. I need to know what money is left, as the team promised the Norwegian authorities that money would be available should further clean-up of the site be necessary in the future ... What I would like to suggest is that we send whatever money is left in the Spitsbergen account to the Governor of Svalbard's Office. The money could be given in trust to the Governor and held for perhaps three years. If no further clean-up is required, the money could then be given to Svalbard Kirke for maintenance of the cemetery ... a suitable donation and thank-you to a community who has undertaken so much on our behalf.' I added that Tom approved of these ideas.

There was, however, no response – nor to a second fax on 27 September. I wrote to the other grant holder, Rob Webster, on 5 October regarding money for the cemetery and the return of Norway's samples. 'We are aware of John Skehel's position that the lab "cannot categorically state that infectious influenza virus is not present," and that "samples can be sent to Norway at any time to a containment 4 lab." John Skehel is only too aware that no BSL 4 lab exists in Norway. In all fairness, the 1998 Longyearbyen meeting should have included a discussion explaining that RT-PCR detection of influenza nucleic acid might be sporadic, and therefore that it would be impossible to state categorically that infectious virus was not present ... Moreover, British HSE regulations should also have been discussed.'

Rob responded on 17 October. 'The funding for the ... project by the

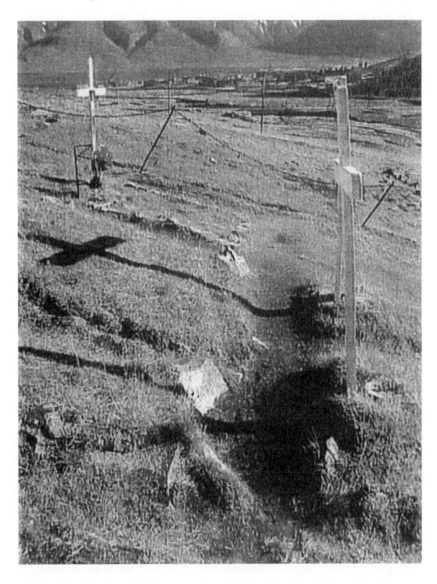

Figure 19   Longyearbyen cemetery, 19 August 2000.

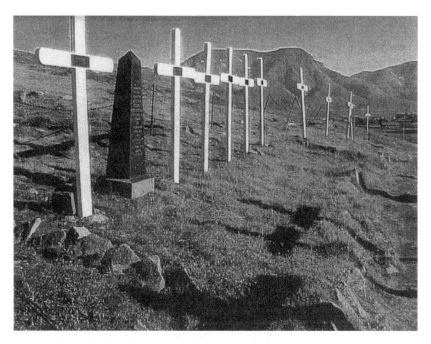

Figure 20   Another view of Longyearbyen cemetery, summer 2000.

National Institutes of Health was completely expended on the project, and there is no carry over money. NIH budgets are carefully monitored in order to insure compliance and the money was spent on the above project. I am delighted to hear from Alan Heginbottom that the site in Svalbard is in outstanding condition. This speaks strongly to Alan Heginbottom's site management.' On the analysis front, 'I understand from Sir John Skehel and Rod Daniels that the resolution of sequence from the samples in London is moving slowly, and it will be a long time before information is available. Hopefully the Canadian laboratory will be able to contribute to the sequence analysis of samples. It would be truly wonderful if the project can contribute to our resolution of knowledge concerning the 1918 influenza pandemic. Thank you for your major role in the project.'

On 20 October, I again faxed John Oxford about clean-up: 'Further to my [three] letters ... I need to know what money is left from our Norwegian expedition.'

Tom did not appreciate John's ignoring my requests. As a result, he wrote two faxes to a Norwegian colleague who was collaborating with John, in the hope that his friend might force John's hand. I refaxed my initial letter of 15 September to John Oxford on 30 October. This latest fax prompted a telephone message from John's assistant, explaining that they had responded to me repeatedly, and a fax, received 31 October (dated 3 October), from John Oxford: 'Pat Meeking assures me that the reserve is held safely by Queen Mary & Westfield College and amounts to £4,567.56. The account has been audited by the College last October and will be audited again next week by external auditors. I have thought carefully about your two ideas. However, I would plan to keep the money in tact at QMW for another 2 years. A very beneficial use would then be something directly to do with the virology or molecular biology of the samples.'

I responded on 5 November:

Thank you for your letter of October 31st, 2000. I am not sure why I did not receive your earlier responses of October 3rd, 14th, or 26th, as my fax number has not changed since August of 1997, and my telephone number and fax number appear in the top right-hand corner of each fax that I send.

Thank you for providing me with the balance ... I am sure that you will appreciate that we must now open the topic of the clean-up of the cemetery to the entire SAG, as the SAG previously decided that the remaining monies in our joint grant would be used for the restoration of the cemetery.

I would like to be pro-active about the clean-up, as there is always the possibility for changes in the grave areas of the seven Spanish flu victims. I think we must consider two scenarios: (1) the six men were interred at 0.5 m; or (2) the men were interred at 2.0 m, and the coffins have been rising since burial. If the latter is true, there is the possibility that the coffins will surface in the future, despite the team's best efforts (namely, exposing only half the coffin) to prevent such an eventuality. If the coffins do surface, it would be better to have the money in Norway.

I think we must also take into consideration climate change. The Intergovernmental Panel on Climate Change (IPCC), the world's foremost authority on the subject, has recently predicted a ... rise in global mean temperature by 2100 AD [1.4–5.8°C]. Such a change may not seem significant. But a temperature decrease of 2.0–4.0°C is enough to bring on a near hemispheric ice age. Warming at the Poles moreover will be much greater than for the Earth as a whole.

Warming will profoundly affect the Earth, causing sea levels to rise, and glaciers and permafrost to melt. Should the thermal regime in Long-yearbyen be altered, the miners' bodies could float to the surface of the cemetery. Climate change is not many years away. The 1980's and 1990's are the warmest decades on record.

I would be grateful if all members of the SAG would consider my points, and respond in writing to me as soon as possible.

Tom wrote on 6 November: 'I agree with your proposal that the moneys be transferred to the local church with proviso that the responsibility of the grave yard is transferred to them.'

John Oxford responded the same day: 'I see no reason what so ever following your fax of November 5th to change from our previous position ie. the balance of the QMW grant will remain at QMW for the next years and should there be no problem at this site the grant should be used for scientific research into the project. A principal grant holder is not allowed to donate a university's money given for research to a charity, however sympathetic we may be. We should be very cautious. As far as I can see the amount of money we have would in no way cope with major issues of floating. In a sense this is a problem for the globe and not our small team.' If the team became 'pro-active,' 'costing could reach tens of thousands of pounds and I suspect all those persons who individually signed and those institutions who signed the original memorandum could be financially responsible. I hope the correspondence on this issue will now close because, as you can imagine, my laboratory move is taking up quite a lot of my time.'

I responded to John the same day: 'Thank you for your response ... I now have four responses: yours and three positive responses. Unfortunately, discussion amongst the SAG does not close upon your request. I will await responses from the two members, who have not responded. As previously decided, I will await responses for only one week, i.e. November 12th. If I have no response, I must assume that the remaining members are in agreement with the proposals.' I clarified my position in response to his remarks. 'Our giving money to Svalbard Kirke would not be a charitable donation, but trust money for repair of the cemetery which we disturbed. It is important to remember that the grant money was previously spent on Arctic clothing and alcohol. It is now time to use the remaining money for upkeep of the cemetery. We must, of course, be pro-active regarding repair work, just as we were pro-active regarding biosafety. The clean-up is part of the science, and the money was ear-marked for restoration.'

Alan responded on 7 November: 'Your proposal to send a sum of money to Svalbard to cover any restoration costs in the future is a legitimate strategy, provided an appropriate and willing recipient can be found ... Any handover of funds would have to be accompanied by an exchange of letters which would clearly show all responsibility is being transferred along with the funds; without this, there is no point doing it. My view is that the situation with the cemetery is very encouraging, but that it is too early for us to regard the site restoration phase as being fully complete.' I agreed with all of Alan's comments. It was necessary, however, before beginning negotiations, to have John Oxford agree to release the money.

Sir John Skehel responded negatively on 9 November: 'I have read the correspondence between you and John Oxford and think his plans to hold the remaining part of the grant in trust at QMW for a couple of years seem appropriate. I am sure we all agree that our promises regarding the site should be completely upheld and we should make sure if and when it needs attention we have sufficient resources to fix it.' There were three (Tom Bergan, Alan Heginbottom, and I) for the proposals, and three (John Oxford, Sir John Skehel, and Rob Webster) opposed. The money would therefore stay at John Oxford's college, and the team would respond to any need for future clean-up rather than being proactive about restoration. However, the team was prepared to cover costs should further repair work become necessary. I had kept my final promise to Norway.

Conclusion: Promises Kept

I still run the project, which I began over nine years ago, which aims to discover the genetic code of the 1918 Spanish influenza virus from tissues of six miners buried in the frozen soils of Svalbard, Norway. I have kept my promises to Norway, my team, and to Canada. The project was run safely and ethically.

The preceding history is first and foremost my story. It is my journey, from my initial desire to search for the elusive causative agent, through finding victims buried in the permafrost, to obtaining permission from the Norwegian authorities to excavate and exhume the bodies in a safe and respectful manner. The frozen tissue, when retrieved, could contain infectious virus, and the unearthing could disturb living descendants of the young miners and the nearby community of Longyearbyen.

My obtaining permission required patience, promises, diplomacy, numerous government approvals, and, of course, financial resources. But, above all, I had to build relationships with the people of Longyearbyen – the citizens, from the owner of the grocery store to the children of Longyearbyen Skole, health care professionals, the pastor, the congregation of Svalbard Kirke, and the family of the young man who froze to death just metres from his home and was buried in the same row as the miners.

The preceding chapters also tell the story of the difficulties faced and overcome in mounting the expedition to retrieve the precious samples: developing detailed excavation plans, applying for the all-important funding, producing the required public relations strategy, and hammering out biosafety protocols to be approved by Norway and the National Institutes of Health in the United States.

The chapters also include surprises. For example, while the team planned carefully for the expedition, Dr Jeffrey Taubenberger, a member of our research team, worked without our knowledge with another researcher, Dr Johan Hultin, who journeyed to Alaska to exhume victims of the 1918 Spanish influenza.

And the pages reveal a key challenge: lobbying for a laboratory agreement, which would have ensured the return of samples to Norway and ultimately would have protected all team members and institutions.

What are the preliminary results? We appear to be getting answers to the long-unanswered puzzle. We appear to have found fragments of the 1918 Spanish flu virus in our tissue samples.

We seem to have new information, never before known about the 1918 virus. For the first time, short fragments of the virus have been recovered from the lung, liver, kidney, and brain. In the past, fragments had been found only in the lung. Our work suggests that the disease may have gone systemic in some cases; in other words, the virus may have attacked numerous organs, not just the lungs, as previously shown.

Our sequencing results are different from those of Dr Taubenberger and Ms Ann Reid in the United States and may suggest that the 1918 pandemic involved more than one virus.

These early results will, however, require independent confirmation by other laboratories. And so the analyses continue today in Britain and in Canada. Norway is still waiting for its samples, which it will use for bacteriological studies.

I am hopeful that the relationship between Spanish flu and encephalitis lethargica will be fully explored. The cause of the latter has not been determined, but anecdotal evidence links it to the preceding 1918 influenza pandemic. I had wanted to test the connection since day one, but the team was not interested.

The scientists at the Windsor Workshop (23–24 August 1996) knew that Baron Constantin von Economo discovered the first case of encephalitis lethargica long before the 1918 influenza pandemic began and therefore argued that the two could not be related. (It has been suggested that a report of epidemic bronchitis of 'high lethality' in an army camp in France in 1917 may, in fact, have been the first indication of the later influenza pandemic.[1]) Moreover, they argued that the neurological disease reached a climax in 1925, years after the influenza pandemic, and that therefore influenza could not be responsible for it. (Neurological sequelae may develop six years or longer following an initial infection of measles.[1])

However, antigens of the influenza A viral strains WSN and NWS have been shown in the brains of six victims of encephalitis lethargica, and researchers Ravenholt and Foege[2] have listed numerous reasons why the two diseases may be linked.

Is there a connection? Only future research will tell. Our attempting isolation of virus or viral genome from the respiratory tract and brains of the miners may shed light on the problem.

This book recounts the story of assembling a large team of experts – medical personnel, safety experts, excavators, microbiologists, and virologists – from Canada, England, Norway, and the United States, and the challenges in leading a team. Many members of the team do not speak the same scientific language and perceive their own academic discipline to be the most important of all the team's various fields of study. Speaking with one team voice is at times difficult, if not impossible, as members separated by thousands of kilometres may sometime negotiate and grant interviews while their colleagues remain unaware.

Leading a team of established, internationally renowned scientists, who do not always work well together and may even be competing with one another, can be challenging. The team provides the backdrop for a glimpse into behaviour when stakes are perceived as high.

It is important in reviewing references and interviewing scientists for a particular task or job to choose people who can work together and who show a high level of personal responsibility. Team members must be able to promote teamwork, keep others informed, listen to and appreciate colleagues, encourage the development of new ideas and techniques, encourage others to express and defend their views, work towards common goals, and align their goals with those of the team.

It is also important to prepare and implement an agreement outlining what is expected from team members in terms of scientific achievements and what the scientists can expect in return – in grants, exposure, and publishing. The agreement should explicitly define reasons for termination.

It is my hope that this book raises questions:

- topical questions regarding public health, such as whether or not we are prepared for the next infectious disease emergency
- ethical questions regarding the nature and practice of science, the rights of subjects, and the rights of the dead
- hierarchical questions, relating to leadership, organizational behaviour, and the relationship among various disciplines.

My voyage is coming to an end after nine years. Before signing off, I find it necessary to summarize what has been achieved. First and foremost, the project focused attention on Spanish flu, which today serves as a useful model for the potential ramifications of an infectious disease emergency or a bioterrorist attack. The catastrophic pandemic reminds us that any large-scale emergency involving infectious disease will require mobilization of public health resources and civil infrastructure.

Second, the project also reminds us not that we are immune to the ravages of flu, but rather that we are vulnerable – each year, outbreaks infect 100 million people in the United States, Europe, and Japan – as people tour increasingly, travel more rapidly, and visit many more places than ever before. And, perhaps most important, the project reminds us that we are due for another fatal flu and that we must be prepared.

Third, our research also focused attention on encephalitis lethargica, the scourge of ~1915–30, which claimed or destroyed the lives of 5 million people, and may still be with us. Occasional cases have been reported ever since the 1950s.

Our project has forged strong relationships with the far northern community of Longyearbyen. Friendship among countries fosters understanding and goodwill and might, in this case, promote advancements in science.

Although no formal permission process existed for exhuming bodies in Norway, the measures required of us by authorities there may serve as a useful model for similar studies. We asked and obtained permission of the families, the town council, the church council, the bishop, the governor of Svalbard, the Norwegian Science Council (in order to ensure inclusion of Norwegian scientists and the upholding of Norwegian scientific standards), the Directorate of Cultural Heritage (as the cemetery is considered a protected historical monument), and state health authorities.

Drawing scientists together from nine disciplines and four countries promoted cross-disciplinary and cross-cultural approaches, which were often new and exciting to individual scientists: for example, exhuming victims in order to determine the genetic code of the 1918 influenza virus was new to the geologists; and using ground-penetrating radar (GPR) to locate graves was a novel approach for the virologists. GPR provides a means of examining what lies beneath the surface of the ground without disturbing precious prehistoric sites and human remains, and may be a useful tool in such disciplines as archaeology and physical anthropology. Destructive excavating and exhuming need be undertaken only if warranted by a GPR study.

Also new were the team's biosafety protocols, relating to exhumation and sampling, decontamination, reburial, and transportation of samples. The Norwegian authorities and the (U.S.) National Institutes of Health approved these protocols, which may serve as a model for similar future research. The American Biological Safety Association invited me to give the Arnold G. Wedum Memorial Lecture for outstanding contributions to biological safety. The team's logistics and excavation plans are also noteworthy, as we shipped seventeen tonnes of material to the Arctic, erected it, and later dismantled it.

The expedition was a success. It was carried out safely and ethically, and it met the conditions of the permission granted, such as protecting the environment, leaving no trace of our work, and practising an open policy with the media.

I am very pleased with and very proud of what our team accomplished. Equally important are Norway's perceptions regarding the project. I know that the authorities there are pleased by the manner in which the project was run, how the expedition and exhumations took place, and how the cemetery is healing.

My last task in the book is to express the team's thanks and my profound gratitude to our host country. The final words of this book are therefore to Norway. Thank you Longyearbyen, thank you Svalbard, thank you Norway.

Epilogue: Update

The first draft of this book was completed in August 2000. As it passed through the hands of referees and editors, more time elapsed, work continued, and I was able to tell the team's story to November 2000. I am now able to extend the history to June 2002.

One of my purposes in writing this volume was to highlight the importance of scientific openness and accountability. What then is the status of the results released to the scientific community and to the media in London in November 1999?

In 2001, NIMR began discussions with Britain's Health and Safety Executive (HSE) to explore the possibility of handling the Svalbard samples at containment level 3. However, the HSE 'did not consider, given the sporadic nature with which we (Daniels et al.) recover PCR-positivity, that the possibility of infectious virus being present in the samples has been exhausted.' As a result, NIMR 'can legally ship samples to Containment 4 laboratories only, unless they have been fixed prior to transport.'

Rod Daniels remained committed to analysing the samples – even hiring a post-doctoral scientist for assistance with PCR – and continued to make progress in sequencing. Daniels reported, 'In attempts to get corroboration of our results we have made two shipments of samples, from autopsies which have yielded PCR positivity in our hands, to the Containment 4 laboratory in Winnipeg. Protocols used at NIMR have been forwarded to the Canadian lab and Rod Daniels spent three weeks in the Canadian lab ... There were some problems in transferring techniques to the Canadian laboratory.'

The Winnipeg lab reported that it was 'not able to confirm the results' but that 'the data generated by Dr. Daniels' group in the U.K.

looked good ... and there is no evidence for contamination.' Winnipeg has ceased to work on the samples.

Daniels reported that, 'given the precautions taken and results of negative controls, it is extremely unlikely that this (contamination) has occurred at the laboratory level ... All work with the Svalbard samples ... has been conducted within the containment 4 laboratory which was newly constructed (1998) in a building remote from the Virology Division where influenza had not been used. All reagents used in the experiment at NIMR were newly designed and bought for the 1918 study.'

As a result, NIMR has once again recommended 'sending the samples to the Taubenberger laboratory.' On 19 June 2002, I suggested that we produce 'a list of researchers/labs who would be able to confirm or refute the results,' as I very much want the issue resolved. However, I strongly oppose exploiting Taubenberger after the team officially severed relations with him. There has yet to be a reply. I hope that answers are forthcoming and that we will publish our results.

Sadly, Tom Bergan passed away in 2001. Prior to his death, Tom asked his life-long friend and colleague Bjorn Berdal to take over his archives of the Svalbard expedition and his influenza-related activities.

I would like to remember Tom Bergan for his courage and scholarly work. Tom joined the expedition in Svalbard a few short weeks after surgery for a disease that he knew would end his life. In our last conversation in Svalbard, and in two later meetings (while Tom was on business) in Toronto, he requested that, in my telling of the story, I make people understand how hard he fought for Norway.

References

Preface

1 Sacks, O. 1973. *Awakenings*. London: Duckworth.

Introduction: A Deadly Killer

1 Crosby, A. 1976. *Epidemic and Peace, 1918*. Westport: Greenwood Press.
2 Collier, R. 1974. *The Plague of the Spanish Lady: The Influenza Pandemic of 1918–1919*. New York: Atheneum.
3 Hill & Knowlton, London. 1998. *The 1918 Project*. London: Hill & Knowlton.
4 Garrett, L. 1995. *The Coming Plague: Newly Emerging Diseases in a World out of Balance*. New York: Penguin Books.
5 Schoch-Spana, M. 2000. Implications of pandemic influenza for bioterrorism response. *Clinical Infectious Diseases* 31: 1409–13.

1 The Spanish Influenza of 1918

1 Durnford, H. (ed.). 1978. *Heritage of Canada: Our Storied Past and Where to Find It*. Montreal: The Reader's Digest Association (Canada) Ltd.
2 Finlay, J., and D. Sprague. 2000. *The Structure of Canadian History*. Don Mills, Ont.: Prentice Hall Ally and Bacon.
3 Francis, R., Jones, R., and D. Smith. 2000. *Destinies: Canadian History since Confederation*. Toronto: Harcourt Canada.
4 Terraine, J. 1968. *The Great War 1914–1918: A Pictorial History*. London: Hutchinson of London.
5 Kulisek, L. 1999. University of Windsor. Personal communication.
6 Trenhaile, A. 1999. University of Windsor. Written communication.

7 Collier, R. 1974. *The Plague of the Spanish Lady: The Influenza Pandemic of 1918–1919*. New York: Atheneum.

8 Pettigrew, E. 1983. *The Silent Enemy: Canada and the Deadly Flu of 1918*. Saskatoon: Western Producer Prairie Books.

9 Beveridge, W. 1977. *Influenza: The Last Great Plague. An Unfinished Story of Discovery.* New York: Prodist.

10 Crosby, A. 1976. *Epidemic and Peace, 1918*. Westport: Greenwood Press.

11 Kumar, P., and M. Clark. 1987. *Clinical Medicine: A Textbook for Medical Students and Doctors*. London: Balliere Tindall.

12 Markham, N. 1986. The north coast of Labrador and the Spanish influenza of 1918. *Them Days* 11 (3): 3–64.

13 Garrett, L. 1995. *The Coming Plague: Newly Emerging Diseases in a World out of Balance*. New York: Penguin Books.

14 Hill & Knowlton, London. 1998. *The 1918 Project*. London: Hill & Knowlton.

15 Phillips, H. 1999. University of Cape Town. Personal communication.

16 Sacks, O. 1973. *Awakenings*. London: Duckworth.

17 Anonymous. 1981. Encephalitis lethargica. *Lancet* 2: 1396–7.

18 Oxford, J. 1999. Is there a link between influenza and encephalitis lethargica? *NeuroScience News* 2 (3–4): 91–2.

19 Christie, A. 1980. Encephalitis lethargica (epidemic encephalitis; Von Economo's Disease). In A. Christie, (Ed.), *Infectious Diseases: Epidemiology and Clinical Practice*. Edinburgh: Churchill Livingstone.

20 Hall, A. 1924. *Epidemic Encephalitis*. Bristol: Wright.

21 Cheyette, S., and J. Cummings. 1995. Encephalitis lethargica: lessons for contemporary neuropsychiatry. *Journal of Neuropsychiatry and Clinical Neurosciences* 7 (2): 125–34.

22 Vitzhum, H., and E. Albert. 1987. Personality change following encephalitis lethargica in childhood. Eventual fate of a patient. *Psychiatr. Neurol. Med. Psychol.* 39 (12): 725–34.

23 Perl, D. 1996. Encephalitis lethargica: the disease and its possible relation to the influenza of 1918. In K. Duncan, (Ed.), *Workshop: The Identification of the 1918 Influenza: August 23–24, University of Windsor, Windsor, Ontario.*

24 BBC Online-QED. 2000. Prisoners of the Forgotten Plague. http://www.bbc.co.uk/qed/sleep.html

25 Clough, C., Plaitakis, A., and M. Yahr. 1983. Oculogyric crises and Parkinsonism. A case of recent onset. *Archives of Neurology* 40 (1): 36–7.

26 Blunt, S., Lane, R., Turjanski, N., et al. 1997. Clinical features and management of two cases of encephalitis lethargica. *Movement Disorders* 12(3): 354–9.

27 Casals, J., Elizan, T., and M. Yahr. 1998. Postencephalitic Parkinsonism – a review. *Journal of Neural Transmission* 105 (6–7): 645–76.

28 Howard, R., and A. Lees. 1987. Encephalitis lethargica: a report of four recent cases. *Brain* 110 (1): 19–33.

29 Maurizi, C. 1989. Influenza caused encephalitis lethargica (e.l.): the circumstantial evidence and a challenge to the naysayers. *Medical Hypotheses* 28(2): 139–42.

30 Ravenholt, R., and W. Foege. 1982. 1918 influenza, encephalitis lethargica, and Parkinsonism. *Lancet* 2: 860–4.

2 The Quest, 1992–1994

1 Collier, R. 1974. *The Plague of the Spanish Lady: The Influenza Pandemic of 1918–1919*. New York: Atheneum.

2 Collier, L., and J. Oxford. 1996. *Human Virology: A Text for Students of Medicine, Dentistry, and Microbiology*. Oxford: Oxford University Press.

3 Hill & Knowlton, London. 1998. *The 1918 Project*. London: Hill & Knowlton.

4 Knauth, O. 1976. Ex-Iowan recalls search for flu bug in frozen north. *Des Moines Register*, 24 June 1976.

5 McKee, A. 1993. Retired, University of Iowa. Personal communication.

6 Staff Librarian. 1993. Armed Forces Medical Library. Personal communication.

7 Staff Librarian. 1993. United States National Library of Medicine. Personal communication.

8 Officer. 1993. Armed Forces Epidemiological Board. Personal communication.

9 Staff Librarian. 1993. The Pentagon Library. Personal communication.

10 Staff Librarian. 1993. NIH Library. Personal communication.

11 Map Librarian. 1993. U.S. Geological Survey Library. Personal communication.

12 Heginbottom, A. 1997. Emeritus scientist, Geological Survey of Canada. Personal communication.

13 Geothermal resources in Iceland: the Reykjavik heating and electricity plan. http://www.energy.rochester.edu/is/reyk

14 Arlov, T. 1994. *A Short History of Svalbard*. Oslo: Norsk Polarinstitutt.

15 Holm, K. 1991. *General Information about Longyearbyen and the Surroundings*. Bodo: Esselte Office.

16 Info-Svalbard. 1996. *Svalbard: Spitsbergen*. Longyearbyen: Svalbard Tourist Board and Info-Svalbard.

17 Svalbard Nett. http://www.svalbard.net
18 Sugden, D. 1982. *Arctic and Antarctic: A Modern Geographical Synthesis.* Totowa, NJ: Barnes and Noble Books.
19 Gaarde, R. 1995. Office of the Governor of Svalbard. Written communication.
20 Ahrens, C. 1998. *Essentials of Meteorology: An Invitation to the Atmosphere.* Minneapolis. West Publishing Company.
21 Alan Booth (Director). 1992. *The Northern Lights* (video). Canada: Yellowknife Films.
22 Governor of Svalbard. 1998. *Svalbard: Experience Svalbard on Nature's Own Terms.* Longyearbyen: Info-Svalbard.
23 Mehlum, F. 1990. *The Birds and Mammals of Svalbard.* Oslo: Norsk Polarinstitutt.
24 Grady, W. 1997. *The Quiet Limit of the World: A Journey to the North Pole to Investigate Global Warming.* Toronto: Macfarlane, Walter & Ross.
25 Mork, K. 1994. Longyearbyen Skole. Written communication.
26 Bergan, T. 1999. University of Oslo and Rikshospitalet. Written communication.

3 Beneath the Crosses, 1994–May 1996

1 Melcher, A., Holowka, S., Pharoah, M., et al. 1997. Non-invasive computed tomography and three-dimensional reconstruction of the dentition of a 2,800-year-old Egyptian mummy exhibiting extensive dental disease. *American Journal of Physical Anthropology* 103: 329–40.
2 Jurmain, R., Nelson, H., Kilgore, L., et al. 2000. *Introduction to Physical Anthropology.* New York: Wadsworth Publishing.
3 Primary containment for biohazards: selection, installation and use of biological safety cabinets. http://www.orcbs.msu.edu/biological/bsc/BSC.htm
4 Norwegian Tourist Board. 1996. *Norway: All-Year Travel Directory to a Land of True Beauty.* New York: Norwegian Tourist Board.

4 First Permission, First Workshop, May–August 1996

1 Duncan, K. (Ed.). 1996. *Workshop: The Identification of the 1918 Influenza: August 23–24, University of Windsor, Windsor, Ontario.*
2 BBC Online – Horizon. 1999. Pandemic script. http://www.bbc.co.uk/horizon/pandemictrans. shtml.

5 Archival Samples? CDC Withdraws, August 1996–June 1997

1 McKee, A. 1997. Retired, University of Iowa. Personal communication.
2 Duncan, K. (Ed.). 1997. *Workshop ll: The Identification of the 1918 Influenza Virus: April 8th, 1997, Centers for Disease Control and Prevention, Atlanta, Georgia.*

6 New Members and GPR Preparations, June–October 1997

1 Gladwell, M. 1997. The dead zone. *New Yorker*, 29 Sept.: 52–65.

7 Through the Ground Darkly, October 1997

1 Davis, J., Heginbottom, J., Duncan, K., et al. 1998. *Phase l Field Report: Locating the Graves of Seven Spanish Flu Victims in Longyearbyen Cemetery, Svalbard, Using Ground Penetrating Radar.* Mississauga: Sensors & Software Inc.
2 Davis, L. 1997. Sensors & Software Inc. Personal communication.
3 Sensors & Software Inc. *1996. Ground Penetrating Radar: An Overview.* Mississauga: Sensors & Software Inc.
4 Heginbottom, A. 1997. Emeritus scientist, Geological Survey of Canada. Personal communication.
5 Davis, J., Heginbottom, J., Annan, P., et al. 2000. Ground penetrating radar surveys to locate 1918 Spanish flu victims in permafrost. *Journal of Forensic Sciences* 45 (1): 68–75.

8 Live Virus? October 1997–January 1998

1 Davis, J., Heginbottom, J. Duncan, K., et al. 1998. *Phase l Field Report: Locating the Graves of Seven Spanish Flu Victims in Longyearbyen Cemetery, Svalbard, Using Ground Penetrating Radar.* Mississauga: Sensors & Software Inc.

9 Mill Hill Meeting, February 1998

1 Propst, M. 1999. Office of the State Medical Examiner. Written communication.
2 Gater, B. 1999. Nome Trial Courts. Written communication.
3 Propst, M. 1999. Office of the State Medical Examiner. Written communication.
4 Propst, M. 1999. Office of the State Medical Examiner. Personal communication.

5 Taubenberger, J. 1998. Armed Forces Institute of Pathology. Personal communication.
6 Reid, A., Fanning, T., Hultin, J., et al. 1999. Origin and evolution of the 1918 'Spanish' influenza virus hemagglutinin gene. *Proceedings of the National Academy of Science* 96: 1651–6.
7 Duncan, K. (Ed.). 1998. *Workshop lll: The Identification of the 1918 Influenza Virus: February 3rd, 1998, National Institute for Medical Research, Mill Hill, London.*

11 Scientific Plan, April–June 1998

1 Bergan, T. 1998. University of Olso and Rikshospitalet. Written communication.

15 Face to Face, 16 August–5 September 1998

The details in chapter 15 are from the log books of Dr Charles Smith, Mr Alan Heginbottom, and Dr Kirsty Duncan and from the team's website, www.spanishflu.utoronto.ca

1 Davies, P. 1999. *Catching Cold: 1918's Forgotten Tragedy and the Scientific Hunt for the Virus that Caused it.* London: Michael Joseph.
2 Duncan, K. (Ed.). 1997. *Workshop ll: The Identification of the 1918 Influenza Virus: April 8th, 1997, Centers for Disease Control and Prevention, Atlanta, Georgia.*
3 Duncan, K. (Ed.). 1998. *Workshop lll: The Identification of the 1918 Influenza Virus: February 3rd, 1998, National Institute for Medical Research, Mill Hill, London.*
4 Houghton, J., Filho, L., Callander, B., et al. (Eds.). 1996. *Climate Change – 1995: The Science of Climate Change: Contribution of Working Group l to the Second Assessment Report of the Intergovernmental Panel on Climate Change.* New York: Cambridge University Press.
5 Watson, R., Zinyowera, M., Moss, R., et al. (Eds.). 1996. *Climate Change 1995. Impacts, Adaptations and Mitigation of Climate Change: Scientific-Technical Analyses.* New York: Cambridge University Press.
6 Mortsch, L. 1996. Environment Canada. Personal communication.
7 Ahrens, C. 1998. *Essentials of Meteorology: An Invitation to the Atmosphere.* Minneapolis: West Publishing Company.
8 Watson, R., Zinyowera, M., Moss, R., et al. (Eds.). 1998. *The Regional Impacts*

of Climate Change: An Assessment of Vulnerability. New York: Cambridge University Press.

9 Houghton, J., Ding, Y., Griggs, D., et al. (Eds.). 2001. *Climate Change 2001: The Scientific Basis. Contibution of Working Group 1 to the Third Assessment Report of the Intergovernmental Panel on Climate Change (IPCC).* Cambridge: Cambridge University Press.

10 McCarthy, J., Canziani, O., Leary, N., et al. (Eds.). *Climate Change 2001: Impacts, Adaptation and Vulnerability, Contribution of Working Group 2 to the Third Assessment Report of the Intergovernmental Panel on Climate Change (IPCC).* Cambridge: Cambridge University Press.

11 Koshida, G., and W. Avis. (Eds.). 1997. *The Canada Country Study: Climate Impacts and Adaptation. National sectoral Volume.* Ottawa: Environment Canada.

16 Waiting for Results, November 1998–October 1999

1 Jarvis, A. 1998. A killer calls. *Windsor Star.* 1998.

17 Fighting for Norway, Fighting for Canada, 11–16 November 1999

1 Influenza – Past, Present and Future: Genetics of Virulence and Pathogenecity: 15th & 16th November 1999. Abstracts. London: Retroscreen Virology.

2 Davies, P. 1999. *Catching Cold: 1918's Forgotten Tragedy and the Scientific Hunt for the Virus That Caused It.* London: Michael Joseph.

3 Talaga, T. 1999. Research piracy storm rages over discovery of flu's 'holy grail.' *Toronto Star.* 14 Nov. 1999.

4 Talaga, T. 1999. One more clue: more than one virus could have caused 1918 flu that killed millions, researchers discover. *Toronto Star.* 16 Nov. 1999.

5 Talaga, T. 1999. Canadians finally get credit in probe of deadly 1918 flu. All ends well in fight with British over release of findings. *Toronto Star.* 17 Nov. 1999.

18 Sharing Samples? November 1999–November 2000

1 Davies, P. 1999. *Catching Cold: 1918's Forgotten Tragedy and the Scientific Hunt for the Virus That Caused It.* London: Michael Joseph.

Conclusion: Promises Kept

1 Oxford, J. 1999. Is there a link between influenza and encephalitis lethar-gica? *NeuroScience News* 2 (3–4): 91–2.
2 Ravenholt, R., and W. Foege. 1982. 1918 influenza, encephalitis lethargica, and Parkinsonism. *Lancet* 2: 860–4.

Index